Reflexology For Holistic Therapists

by
Colin Paddon Ph.D., D.Ac., D.N.M.

Reflexology For Holistic Therapists

by
Colin Paddon Ph.D., D.Ac., D.N.M.

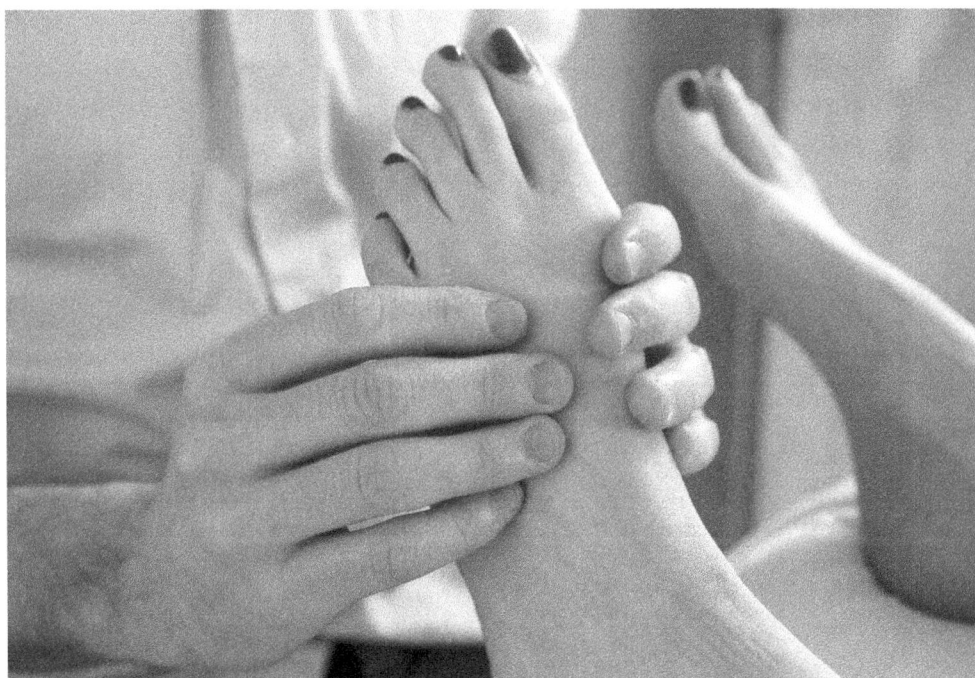

Airmid Holistic Books, Los Angeles

Airmid Holistic Books, Sunland, CA 91040
© Colin Paddon 2009. All rights reserved.
Published 2009.
Printed in the United States of America

ISBN 978-0-9820318-2-7

REFLEXOLOGY COURSE

The following general competencies are those which would be typical of a graduate Reflexologist upon entry into the labour market:

- A qualified Reflexologist can obtain gainful employment in a variety of settings, such as Hair, Beauty or Aesthetic salons, Chiropodist clinics, Holistic Health Clinics, Health spas and fitness clubs, and within the personnel care segments of the entertainment industry.
- A qualified Reflexologist can expect to earn an average of Thirty Dollars to Fifty Dollars per treatment, a treatment would take approximately forty minutes to one hour.

REFLEXOLOGY

DESCRIPTION: To provide a correspondence course of instruction that will allow the student to study fromhome and still become competent in the art and science of Reflexology.

THEORY/SKILL OBJECTIVES:

1. Introduction to Holistic Health Care
2. Legal Aspects of Using Reflexology
3. Health & Hygiene
4. General Anatomy of the Feet
5. The Underlying Causes of Illness
6. Foot Disorders
7. The History of Reflexology
8. Relaxation Methods
9. Systematic Treatment Procedure
10. Case-Studies and Record-keeping
11. Essential Oils and Creams
12. Setting up a Business

TABLE OF CONTENTS

Introduction to Holistic Health Care

HISTORY AND ORIGINS

Holistic healthcare has been used since the beginning of time, but Hippocrates, (pronounced; Hip-poc cra-tees) born in Greece around 460 BC described the effects of 300 plants and their uses, and wrote a treatise on herbal medicine, placing more importance on the moral qualities needed to be a doctor, such as discernment and devotion. To this day Hippocrates is still revered as the " Father of Medicine ", and the "Hippocratic Oath" continues to be taught to medical students today.

Many Greek doctors were employed by Rome as military surgeons.   One of these Greek surgeons was Galen. Born in Pergamon in Asia Minor around 131-199 AD., Galen reworked many of the old Hippocratic ideas, and formalized his theories in medical texts used extensively by the Romans and medieval Arab physicians. He became the physician to the Roman Emperor Marcus Aurelius and served as a surgeon to a school of gladiators. It was recorded that no gladiator died of his wounds during Galen's term of office. Perhaps this is not surprising, since he was familiar with and used several essential oils from which he prepared his remedies. He wrote a great deal on the theory of plant medicine and divided plants into various medicinal categories, which are still known as "Galenic".

The healing knowledge used so extensively by the Egyptians and Greeks greatly influenced theRomans. One of these Roman doctors was the Greek Dioscorides, (pronounced; di-o-scor-ides).Having made a detailed study of the application of plants and aromatics, he compiled an account ofhis works and wrote in 50 AD. five-huge volumes called "De Materia Medica" also known as the Herbarius. This remained the standard text for 1,500 years, in which he gave a detailed account of the healing properties of many herbs. This was later translated into Persian, Hebrew, Anglo-Saxon and many other languages.

980-1037 AD. Ali-Ibn Sina, known to us as Avicenna (pronounced; Av-vi-seen-na) the Arab, wrotebooks on the properties of over 800 plants and their effects on the human body.

Knowledge of herbal medicine gained during the Crusades in the Middle East and Islands of the Mediterranean was disseminated throughout Western Europe by the Knights and their armies.   Not only did they bring back the actual plants and the knowledge of how use them, but also the different healing methods they employed.

9

During the Bubonic Plague in the 17th century, frankincense and pine were burned in the streets. Indoors, incense, perfumed gums and resins were worn around the neck. During the Black Death era, aromatics were the best antiseptics available. Exactly how effective these measures were, can only be surmised. History reported that those in closest contact with aromatics especially the perfumers, were virtually immune. Since all aromatics are antiseptic it is likely that some of those used were indeed effective protection against the plague.

Until the 19th century, medical practitioners carried a small cassoulet filled with aromatics on top of their walking sticks. This acted as a personal antiseptic, and would be held up to the nose when visiting anycontagious patients.

In the Middle Ages, many herbal books were written in Latin. In his 16th century writings William Turner, The Father of Botany was the first to describe herbs and their medicinal properties inEnglish and thus helping to popularize herbal medicine. His motive in doing this was to assist the apothecaries and common folk that gathered herbs to help them understand which plants physicians wrote about in prescriptions. This action earned both himself and Nicholas Culpepper the wrath of the newly formed College of Physicians, because it allowed ordinary people to find herbal medicines in the hedgerows and fields instead of paying vastly inflated apothecaries' bills.

In 1653 Nicholas Culpepper wrote his book "Complete Herbal" . In the 18th century, essential oils were used widely in medicines. Salmon's dispensary of 1896 contains many aromatic remedies. The 19th century found that many essential oils could be produced synthetically. This was a much cheaper and easier process than using natural plants.

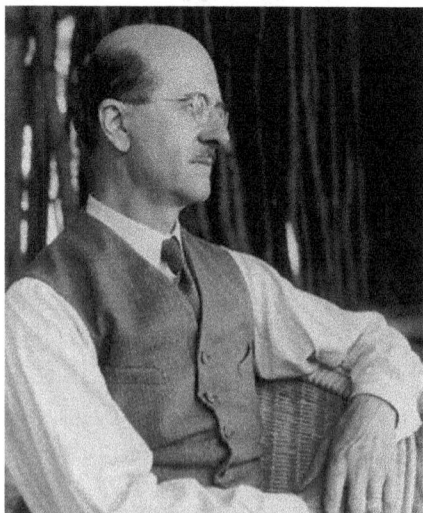

"Rene-Maurice Gattefosse" A French chemist workingin his family's perfumer business, coined the term"Aromatherapy" in his book entitled "Aromatherapie" which was published in 1928. During this time he was investigating the antiseptic properties of essential oils. He also re-discovered the healing properties of lavender. Two things happened which helped to extend this interest in aromatic essential oils. Firstly, cosmetics often contained antiseptics and he discovered that essential oils had greater antiseptic properties than some of the antiseptic chemicals of the time. Secondly, one of Gattefosse's hands was badly burned when a small explosion occurred in his laboratory during an experiment. He instantly immersed it in neat essential oil of lavender, and was only partly surprised when he found that the burn healed at a phenomenal rate,with no sign of infection, and leaving no scar.

He also found that many essential oils when used in their entirety were more effective than using asynthetic substitutes or their isolated active ingredients. For instance, the active ingredient in eucalyptus is called "eucalyptol" or "cineol". The antiseptic properties are more active when used as a whole plant in its natural form and react stronger than when separated or isolated. Which is why we also use Aromatherapy essential oils in the treatment of the feet with reflexology.

Legal Aspects of Using Reflexology

QUALIFICATIONS

To become qualified in Reflexology means that you must have attended a school or completed a correspondence course that meets the requirements of the governing body in power at the present moment. Most schools offer qualifications after you have rigorously been tested in your knowledge of the modality, its history and methods as well as the actual treatment. Also it's important to understand the contra-indications, when not to treat is as important as when to treat. Most schools offer a curriculum that covers the requirements for certification that include, anatomy & physiology, some pathology and Reflexology theory and practice, health & hygiene, and legalities. Before embarking on the course you have chosen, check to see if your school is registered as a private or vocational school, who endorses or recognises their training and how long have they been in business as well as the qualifications and years of teaching experience the instructor has. Once satisfied, enjoy your learning experience and put it to use immediately.

INSURANCE

It is impossible to obtain insurance coverage if you have no qualifications. What insurance do you need? There are two areas that need addressing: Personal malpractice and Liability insurance

1. Personal malpractice: Personal malpractice is a prerequisite for all and any health care practitioner and in most area's it is mandatory. Personal malpractice will offer you protection if you become involved in a lawsuit due to neglect or professional misconduct. We are living in an age where lawsuits are becoming more common and so it would behove you to protect your self and your loved ones from thistype of attack.

    One of the most common questions is whether to get one million or two million dollars of coverage. You will only need one million if you are operating a small practice and morecoverage will be needed if your practice grows or you wish to practice in a public facility like a hospital.

2. Liability insurance
    Public liability insurance is only needed if you are practising in your own premises in case a person falls or hurts themselves whilst at your home for instance. If you work for someone else at their premises then its their responsibility to acquire this insurance, as it's the building that's insured not you.

On an additional note: It would also benefit you to belong to an association, not that this association will offer you value for money, but it does offer assistance in case of trouble or if you have questions or need support. Other than that, they tend to demand more than they are willing to give, so chose carefully before committing you resources.

Health & Hygiene

IMPORTANCE OF HYGIENE

The Importance of hygiene cannot be over emphasised, your livelihood depends on your ability to be discerning, if you catch an unpleasant disorder or give one, you can imagine what I'm saying. Would you go to a premises that appeared dirty or unsanitary? Would you revisit a therapist that had dirty hands or nails? No I believe you would not. Body odour is another concern for both you and your client. There are a few simple rules to follow that will help you to avoid the problems that may come back to haunt you later in life.

1. Always wash you hands before and after each treatment with antiseptic/antibacterial soap.

2. Always wash the feet you are about to work on with antiseptic/antibacterial soap or better yet offer them a foot bath and soak the feet in a solution of antiseptic/antibacterial soap or Ti-Tree essential oil.

3. Inspect the feet throughly for warts, cuts and bruises and athletes foot and fungal infections.

4. Never touch your face especially near eyes, nose and mouth when working on someone else's feet.

5. Never work on feet with cuts or skin rashes.

6. Never work on feet if you have any cuts on your own hands.

7. If in doubt, don't do it. That means if you are not sure if you should be working on this person for whatever reason, don't.

8. Always use dry, clean towels and wear a lab coat or something similar to act as a barrier.

9. If you find nail fungus ask if you can use Ti-Tree to get rid of it, remember you can contract it if you don't treat it NOW.

10. Never use a tool to treat or replace your own hands, they can harbour germs and spread disorders.

Section six deals with disorders you might come across, so more on this topic later.

HEALTH RISKS
Bacteria

Bacteria (microbes) are microscopic, unicellular organisms that are carried from place to place by humans, animals, insects, food, soil, water and air. Some of them are beneficial to humans (nonpathogenic ie; penicillium), while others are disease producing (pathogenic).

Two factors determine the microbe's strength:
- how quickly it reproduces
- toxigenicity (the strength of its poisons)

It is difficult to destroy bacteria although their growth and reproduction can be controlled bychemicals and natural substances.

Classifications of Pathogenic Bacteria

Compared with a virus, the bacteria is quite large. In one single drop of water, there could be as many as 50 million bacteria.

There are hundreds of different classifications of bacteria.

Pathogenic bacteria are classified into three main groups, according to shape;

1) Cocci

   These are round-shaped organisms which appear singly or in groups as follows:

   a) Staphylococci

   These are pus forming organisms which grow in bunches or clusters, and are present in abscesses, pustules and boils.

   b) Streptococci

   These are pus forming organisms which grow in chains, as found in blood poisoning.

   c) Diplococci

   These grow in pairs, and cause pneumonia.

2) Bacilli

   These are rod-shaped organisms. They are the most common and produce such diseases astetanus (lockjaw), influenza, typhoid, tuberculosis and diphtheria. Many bacilli are spore producers.

3) Spirilla

   These are curved or corkscrew-shaped organisms. They are further subdivided into several groups, of chief importance is the spirochaetal organisms in syphilis.

Growth and Reproduction

These cells are surrounded by a slim layer of varying thickness. This coating protects the cell from unfavourable environmental conditions and allows it to adhere to the surface of its food supply or to another cell or organism. The cell can remain dormant or inactive when conditions for growth are lacking. In other words, when conditions become favourable, this will enable them to enter a period of very rapid growth and reproduction.

Conditions for Growth

    a) Suitable Temperature
- Most bacteria thrive at a temperature of 80-100 degrees F.
- Those causing human infections grow best at 98.6F.

    b) Moisture - active bacterial cells are 90% water. In dry surroundings, water loss will make a cell inactive, eventually resulting in its death. c) Darkness - exposure to sunlight and ultraviolet radiation will kill the cells.

Bacterial Infections

Pathogenic bacteria becomes a menace to health when they invade the body, an infection occurs if the body is unable to cope with the bacteria and their harmful toxins. A local infection is indicated by a boil or pimple containing pus, it is generally located in one specific area. A general infection results when the blood stream carries the bacteria and their toxins to all parts of the body, as in blood poisoning. The presence of pus is a sign of infection, staphylococci are the most common pus-forming bacteria. The following is found in pus; bacteria, waste matter, decayed tissue, body cells and both living and dead blood cells.

Viruses

These are extremely small pathogenic germs which live on living tissue. They gain entrance into body cells and depend on the nutrients inside the cell for all their metabolic needs.

AIDs

AIDS is a virus transmitted through sexual contact or through contact with infected bodily fluids,such as blood. For maximum safety, anyone performing any manual extractions or performing any manual procedure involving body fluids should wear surgical rubber gloves or latex gloves.

Infection Sources
The chief sources of infection are:

      a. unclean hands

      b. unclean implements

      c. open sores and pus

      d. mouth and nose discharges

      e. common use of drinking cups and towels

      f. uncovered coughing and sneezing

Bacteria Enters the Body
There can be no infection without the presence of pathogenic bacteria. Pathogenic bacteria mayenter the body by way of:

      a. a break in the skin, such as a cut, pimple or scratch

      b. breathing (air) or by swallowing (water and food)

      c. the nose (air)

      d. the eyes or ears (dirt)

Body's Response to Infection
The body fights infection by means of its defensive forces, consisting of:

      a. the unbroken skin, which is the body's first defense

      b. body secretions, such as perspiration and digestive juices

      c. white blood cells within the blood that destroy bacteria

      d. antitoxins that counteract the toxins produced by bacteria

The Body's Defences

The body is constantly defending itself against invasion by disease. its defences are called first, second and third-line defences.

First-Line Defences

Bacteria can enter the body through any orifice, such as the mouth, nose, etc. Bacteria are takeninto the body in food and liquids, and can enter by way of injuries that cut, break, or puncture the skin. Healthy skin is one of the body's most important defences against disease. It acts as a barrier by resisting the penetration of harmful bacteria.

The nose has mucous and fine hairs that serve as a protection against bacteria. When a person sneezes or coughs, the body is reacting to protect itself against bacteria. Other barriers are juices in the stomach, and the organisms within the intestines and other areas of the body. Tears in the eyes also serve to flush out harmful bacteria and foreign objects.

Second-Line Defence

The body also defends itself from harmful bacteria by producing inflammation, redness and swelling, reveal an increase in temperature and metabolic activity. The inflamed area will be sensitive to the touch. The white blood cells go into action to destroy harmful microorganisms in the bloodstream and tissues so that healing can take place.

Third-Line Defence

The body can produce substances which can inhibit or destroy harmful bacteria. These protective substances are the anti-bodies.

As a Reflexologist you must not perform a service on any client who has a contagious disease. To avoid the spread of disease, keep yourself and your surroundings clean.

Keep everything you come into contact with clean. See that everything you use is clean before each use, and sanitized. Many clients will make an impression solely, and rightfully based upon the cleanliness of a salon. You must be aware of the importance of personal hygienic living, eating healthful and nourishing foods, getting proper rest, exercise and having physical check-ups in order to maintain your health.

Contra-indications

1. Open wounds

2. Infectious diseases or disorders

3. Excessive bruising

TREATMENTS

Systematic Procedures

Always work systematically from the top of the foot to the bottom or heel, never jump from one point to another, make the movements flowing and gentle, but firm.

3 Golden Rules of Reflexology

It must look good. It must feel good. It must do good.

Foot Diagnostics

Carefully check the feet for contagious disorders and skin breaks or bruises.

Reflexology Charts

Know your reflex points by heart, you must know what point your working on.

Differences Between Treatments and Assessments

When you treat the foot, you stay on a tender area and work gently, slowly increasing the firmness, until you are back to full pressure and the client is still feeling comfortable.

Foot Care

Wash the feet carefully and gently (as if they were asleep and you did not wish to wake them). Use warm water and an antiseptic (like an essential oil) as well as something to help the foot relax that smells good (like essential oil of peppermint).

General Anatomy of the Feet

INTRODUCTION

The following notes are subject matter relating to the amount of knowledge needed to become a therapist. Should you feel that further study would prove beneficial, then by all means feel free to do so. However, the course level of knowledge examination will be taken from material provided.

This book makes no pretence at enveloping the whole subject of anatomy and physiology, but is aimed at giving you the student a basic understanding of related anatomical parts, position and function.

Anatomy is defined as the study of the structure of the body. Physiology is defined as being the study of the function of those parts.

For example:
- The heart weighs approx. nine ounces, is pear shaped and lies two-thirds on the left-hand side of the chest area and one third to the right. That is the basic anatomy.
- The heart pumps blood around the body after first oxygenating it via the lungs. That is the basic physiology.

By combining the knowledge of anatomy and physiology, we are able to get a clearer picture of the organ and its relationship to the body, together with its form and composition, and so, improve ourunderstanding of the body as a whole.

For simplicity, the body will be divided into eight main systems. Some text books divide or subdivide into more or less systems, however, for the purpose of this course we shall look at them as follows:

1.	The Skeletal System:	Bones, structure, support, articulation and mobility.
2.	The Muscular System:	Two types of muscle, voluntary and involuntary muscles and ligaments.
3.	The Vascular System:	Including the lymphatic system, heart and blood vessels.
4.	The Neurological System:	Covers most of the nerves of the body and brain.
5.	The Digestive System:	Including related organs of digestion.

6.	The Respiratory System:	Lungs.
7.	Genito-Urinary System:	Including the reproductive and kidney system.
8.	The Endocrine System:	The glands and their effects on the body.

All professional therapists should have a basic knowledge of medical terminology, which you will need to become familiar with to assist in understanding other professionals. Although we can not teach all the terms in this short book, those which you will use the most will be taught. Understanding this terminology will make subsequent study that much easier.

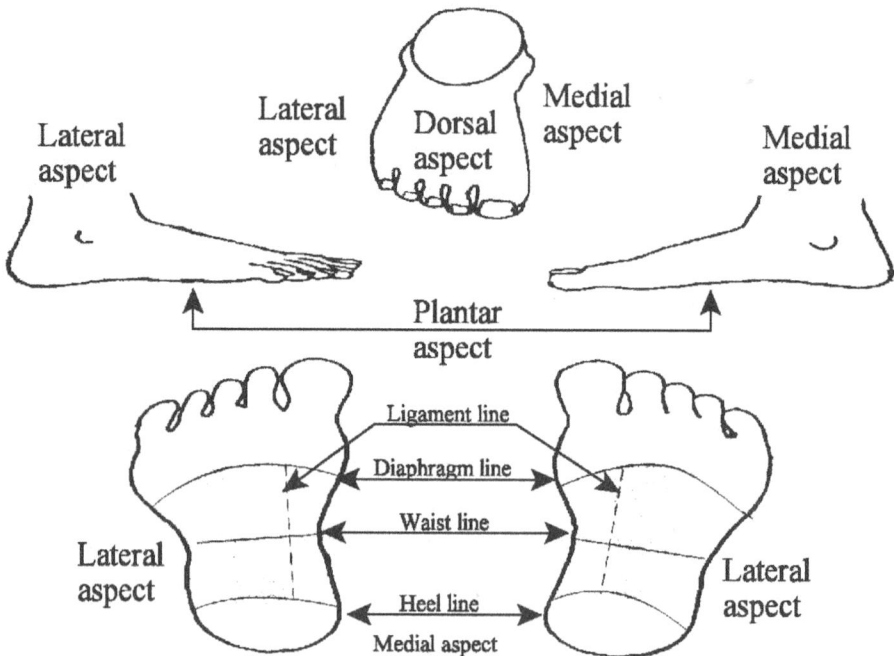

HISTORICAL

It is difficult to trace the exact study of anatomy and physiology, although the Egyptians with their famous embalming process must have gained a lot of knowledge about the human body as they perfected this art. It is interesting to note that the "R" which European doctors write at the top of prescriptions, is in fact the **"R" symbol of the Eye of Horus**, (the hawk headed sun god), who lost his eye in battle and had it restored by Thoth, who was adopted as the patron God of physicians. Thoth was one of the many Gods invoked by ancient Egyptian doctors while administering their remedies.

It was with the Greeks that we learned in detail about anatomy and physiology. The first detailed accounts from this era came from **Hippocrites**, often referred to as the **Father of Medicine**.

Aristotle, is accredited as being the founder of comparative anatomy.

From the Roman era, a vast collection of surgical and dissecting instruments have been unearthed, which indicate a considerable understanding of anatomical form and function.

It was in the second century A.D. that **Galen** lived, and his name is still remembered as being one of the greatest physicians and anatomists of antiquity. His work established the foundation of European anatomy as we know it.

From the sixteenth century medical school in Italy, **Paracelsus Von Hohenheim**, graduated to become a progressive medical teacher and did much to alter the accepted ideas of his day.

In 1543, **Vesalius** published his first drawings of the structure of the human body in his book "Fabric of the Human Body", and so paved the way for modern anatomy.

Since those early times many talented doctors have contributed to expand the knowledge of anatomy in the search to uncover and simplify the complex functions of the human body.

William Harvey is linked to the role and function of the heart and the process of oxygenated blood through the lungs.

Malpighi discovered capillary circulation in 1661.

Avenbrugger of Austria discovered "Percussion" in the middle of the 18th century.

Rene Laennec invented the stethoscope.

1822 **Dr William Beaumont** contributed much to the understanding of the function of the digestive system.

1867 **Lister** discovered the antiseptic principles.

1877 **Pasteur** demonstrated the role of germs and disease.

1895 **Roentgen** discovered X-ray.

1904 **Baylis and Stanley** identified the first hormone.

1912 **Frederick Gowland Hopkins**, discovered vitamins.

1928 **Alexander Fleming** discovered antibiotics (penicillin).

1953 **James Watson and Francis Crick** discovered the double helix of DNA (Dioxyribonucleicacid).

Anatomy and physiology are subjects of continuous study and discovery. Each year will bring new discoveries and understanding.

GENERAL ANATOMY & PHYSIOLOGY

By combining the knowledge of anatomy and physiology, we are able to get a clearer picture of the organ and it's relationship to the body, together with it's form and composition, and so, improve our understanding of the body as a whole.

Functions of the Foot
1. Adapt to ground surfaces to enable the body to maintain balance and stay erect.
2. Helps propel the body in any direction required.
3. Acts as a shock absorber by absorbing most of the pressure that could otherwise cause stress on other joints of the body (ie; knees, spinal column).
4. The feet support the weight of the body.
5. They also stop the ends of the legs from fraying...

Bones of the Foot
Each foot contains 26 small bones with over one hundred ligaments and muscles to help maintain balance and to keep the bones in their correct position as well as to provide elasticity to joints. The main strength in the foot comes from the big toe, while the centre of balance is the ball of the foot. Good foot hygiene and foot care is important because on average, a person can walk more than 70,000 miles in their lifetime. This is equivalent to 3 times around the world.

26 Bones of the Foot
7 tarsal bones (ankle)
5 metatarsal bones (instep bones)
14 phalanges (bones of the toes)

Tarsal bones are composed of:
1 talus
1 calcaneus
1 navicular
1 cuboid
3 cuneiform
Seven bones form the heel and the back part of the instep of the foot.

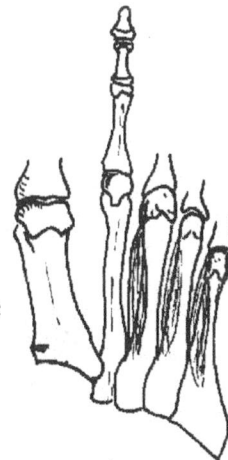

Metatarsal Bones
These five bones form the front part of the instep.

Phalanges

The fourteen phalanges form the bones of the toes. The large toe is composed of two phalanges while the other four toes have three phalange bones. The ball of the foot is the area where the phalanges connect to the underside of the metatarsal bones.

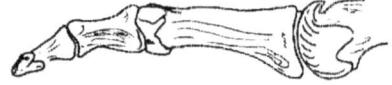

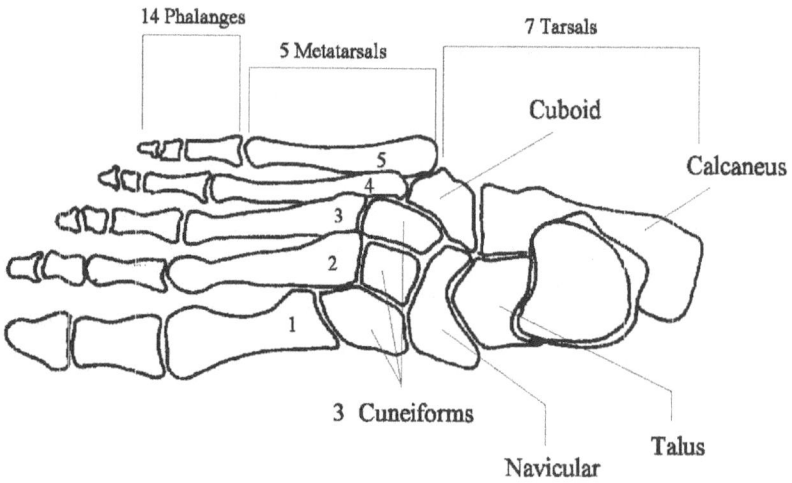

14 Phalanges

5 Metatarsals

7 Tarsals

Cuboid

Calcaneus

5

4

3

2

1

3 Cuneiforms

Navicular

Talus

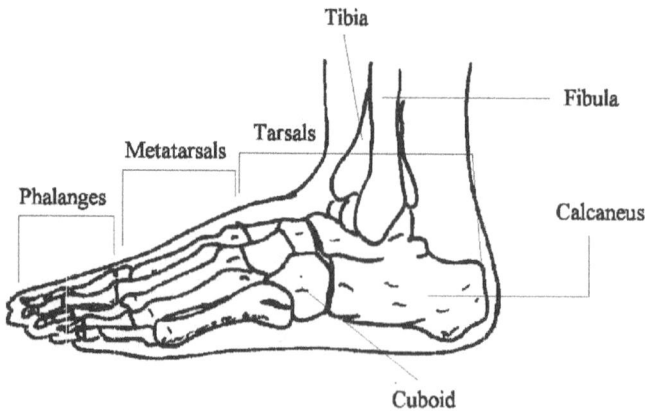

Tibia

Fibula

Tarsals

Metatarsals

Phalanges

Calcaneus

Cuboid

Bones of the foot and lower extremities...

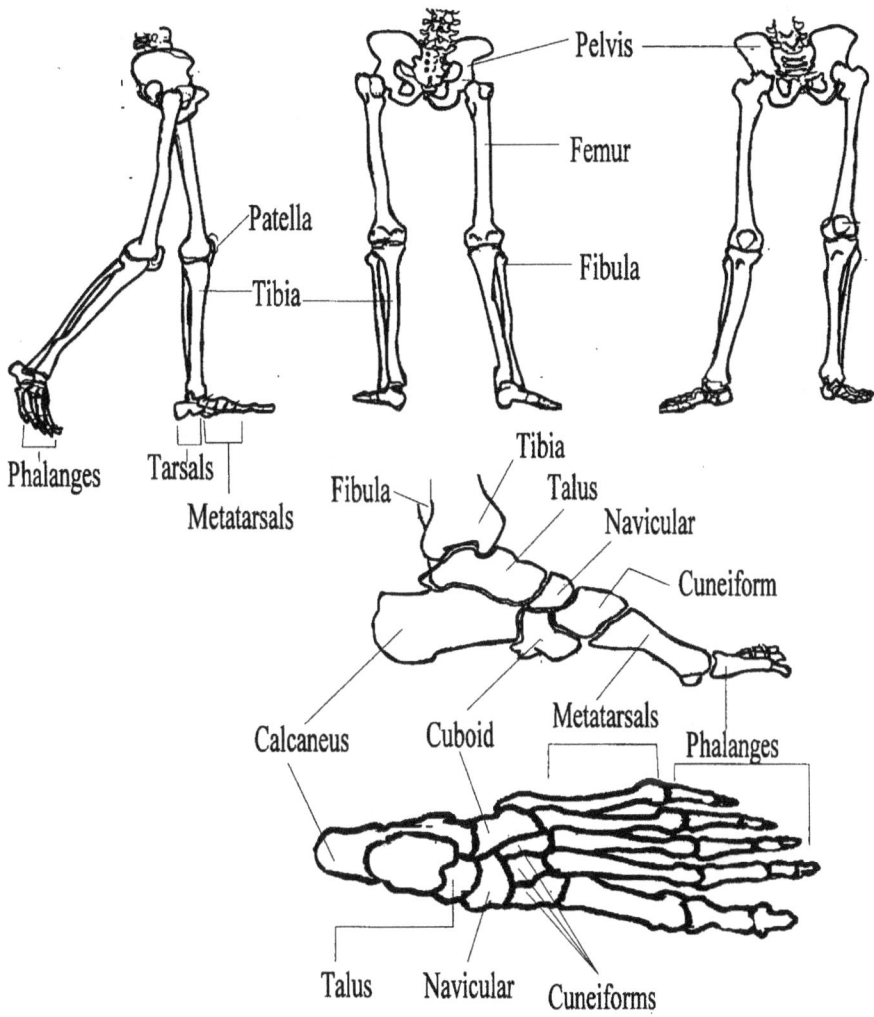

Patella

Tibia

Phalanges   Tarsals

Metatarsals

Pelvis

Femur

Fibula

Tibia

Fibula   Talus

Navicular

Cuneiform

Calcaneus   Cuboid   Metatarsals

Phalanges

Talus   Navicular   Cuneiforms

The Arch

The metatarsal and tarsal bones of the foot combine together to form **three arches. Two arches run lengthwise, and one arch runs crosswise (transverse).**

1. One lies on the inside part of the foot and is called the **Medial Longitudinal Arch.**
2. While the other lies along the outer edge of the foot and is named the **Lateral Longitudinal Arch**. These longitudinal arches run from the heel, to the connection point of the metatarsal and the phalanges. Both longitudinal arches press down on the ground at the heel and the ball of the foot, this prevents any jarring action that might possibly shock the spinal cord. A thick layer of flexible cartilage covers the end of the bones of the arches, it helps to make them shock absorbent.
3. The third arch lies in the metatarsal region and extends across the ball of the foot and is called the **Transverse or Metatarsal Arch**. Arches strengthen the foot and provides flexibility and the natural elastic spring of the foot, especially in activities such as walking and jumping.

Strong ligaments and tendons hold the bones of the foot in their arched positions. However, the arches may fall due to weakness in these ligaments and tendons. The constant pressure of the body slowly flattens them causing *"flat feet"*. With these fallen arches, there may be pain, some of the factors that contribute to this condition are; dietary or hormonal imbalance, poor posture, being overweight and improperly fitted shoes.

Ligaments and Muscles of the Foot

Ligaments and muscles support the arches of the foot. The long plantar ligament is very strong. it keeps the bones of the foot in place and protects the nerves, muscles and blood vessels in the hollow of the foot. The foot has as many muscles as the hand. However, its structure permits less flexibility and freedom of movement than does that of the hand.

Tough thick skin covers the sole of the foot, a thick pad of fatty tissue lies beneath the skin, the bones and the plantar ligament. This layer of fat acts like an air cushion to protect the inner parts of the foot from pressure and jarring.

Nerves of the Foot
Tibial

Supplies the extensor and flexor muscles of the foot and toes as well as the skin of the sole and the dorsum of the foot.

Common Peroneal Nerve
Runs beneath the head of the Fibula and then divides into the deep Peroneal and the Superficial Peroneal Nerves.

Deep Peroneal (Anterior Tibial)
Supplies the extensor muscles of the foot and the toes and the skin of the dorsum of the foot.

Superficial Peroneal   (Musculocutaneous)
Supplies the peroneal muscles and the skin of the external part of the lower leg and foot.

Dorsal Cutaneous (Intermedial and Lateral)
Supplies the top of the foot.

Plantar Nerve (Lateral and Medial)
Supplies the sole of the foot as well as the deep muscles of the foot and toes.

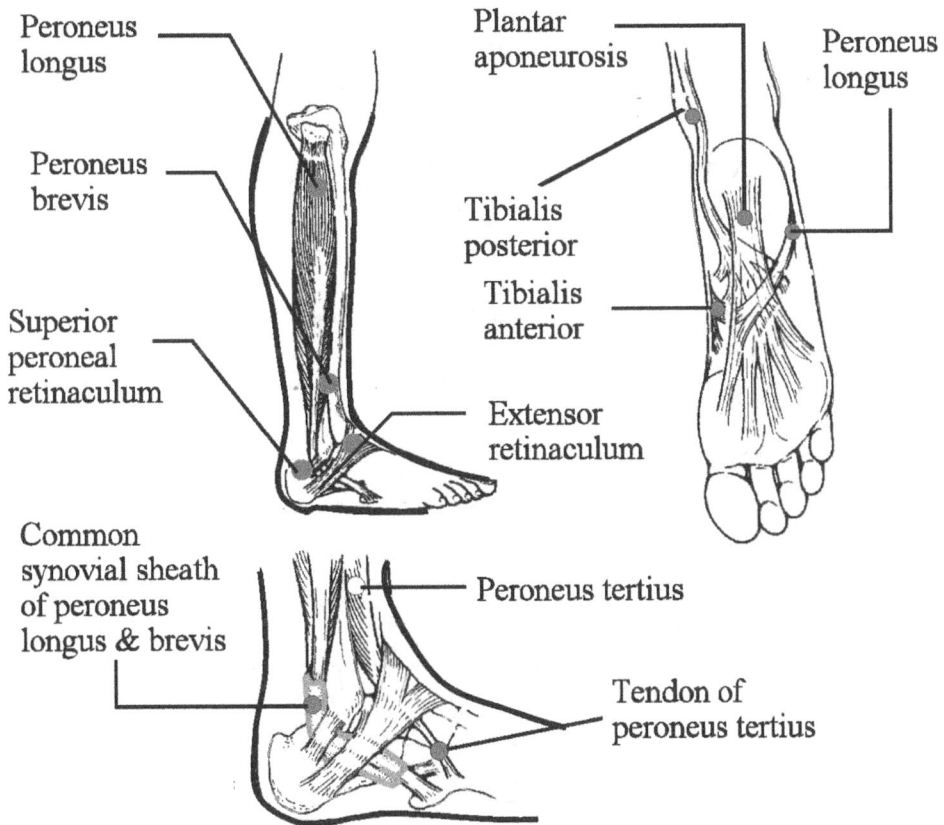

Peroneus longus

Peroneus brevis

Superior peroneal retinaculum

Common synovial sheath of peroneus longus & brevis

Plantar aponeurosis

Tibialis posterior

Tibialis anterior

Extensor retinaculum

Peroneus longus

Peroneus tertius

Tendon of peroneus tertius

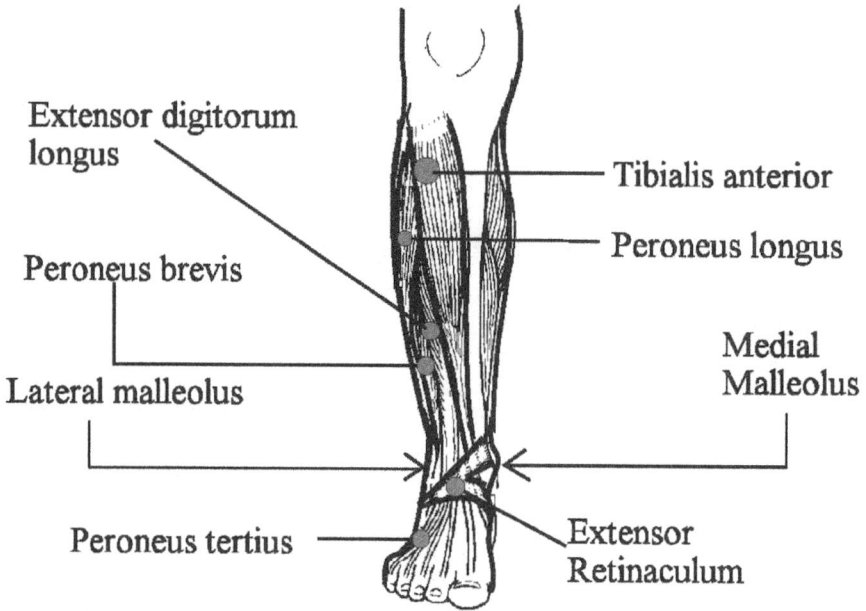

Extensor digitorum longus

Tibialis anterior

Peroneus longus

Peroneus brevis

Medial Malleolus

Lateral malleolus

Peroneus tertius

Extensor Retinaculum

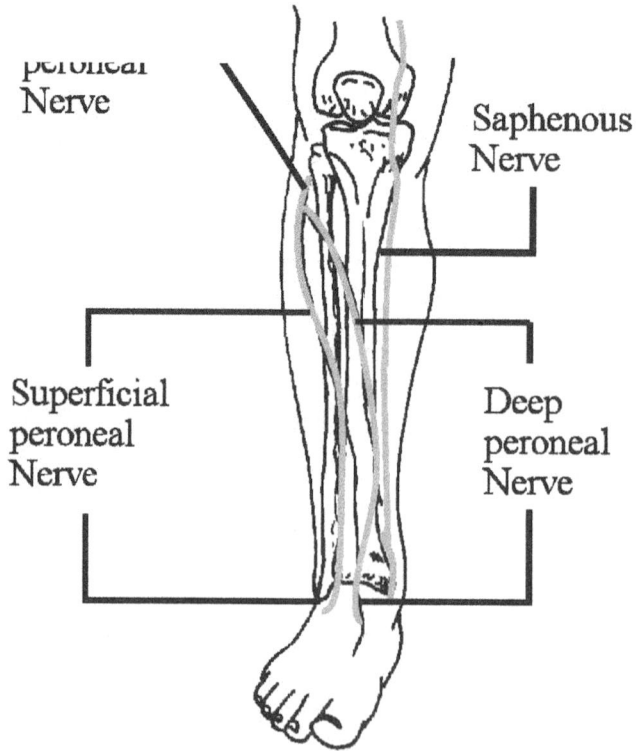

peroneal Nerve

Saphenous Nerve

Superficial peroneal Nerve

Deep peroneal Nerve

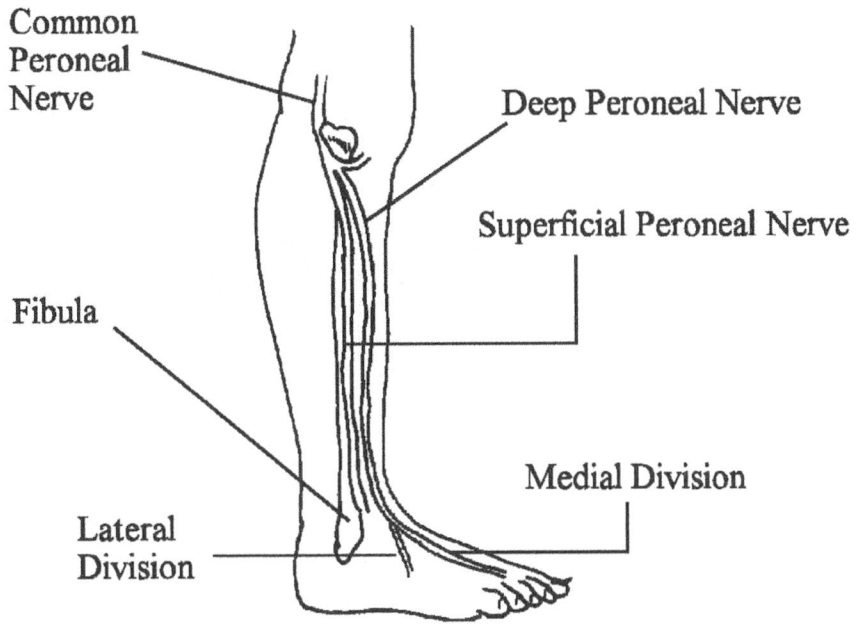

Common Peroneal Nerve

Deep Peroneal Nerve

Superficial Peroneal Nerve

Fibula

Medial Division

Lateral Division

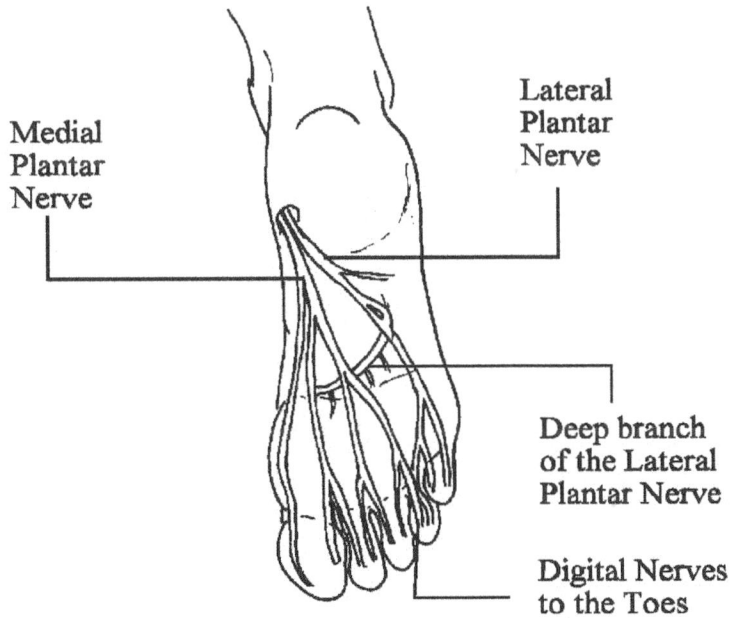

Medial Plantar Nerve

Lateral Plantar Nerve

Deep branch of the Lateral Plantar Nerve

Digital Nerves to the Toes

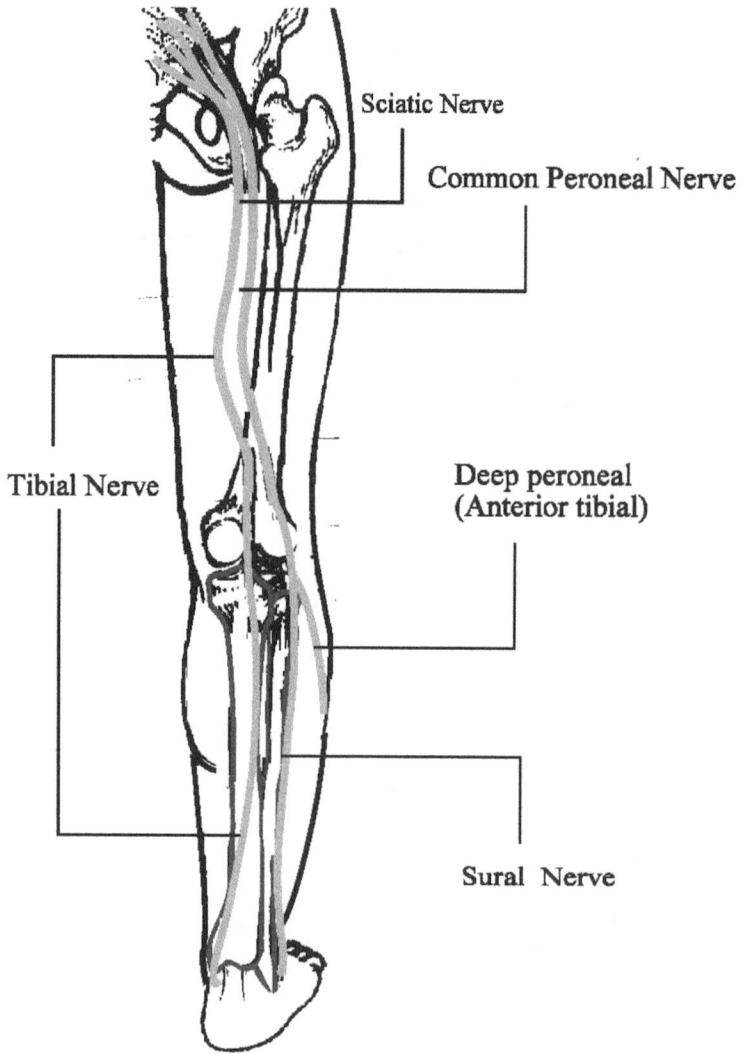

Sciatic Nerve

Common Peroneal Nerve

Tibial Nerve

Deep peroneal
(Anterior tibial)

Sural Nerve

UNDERSTANDING LYMPH

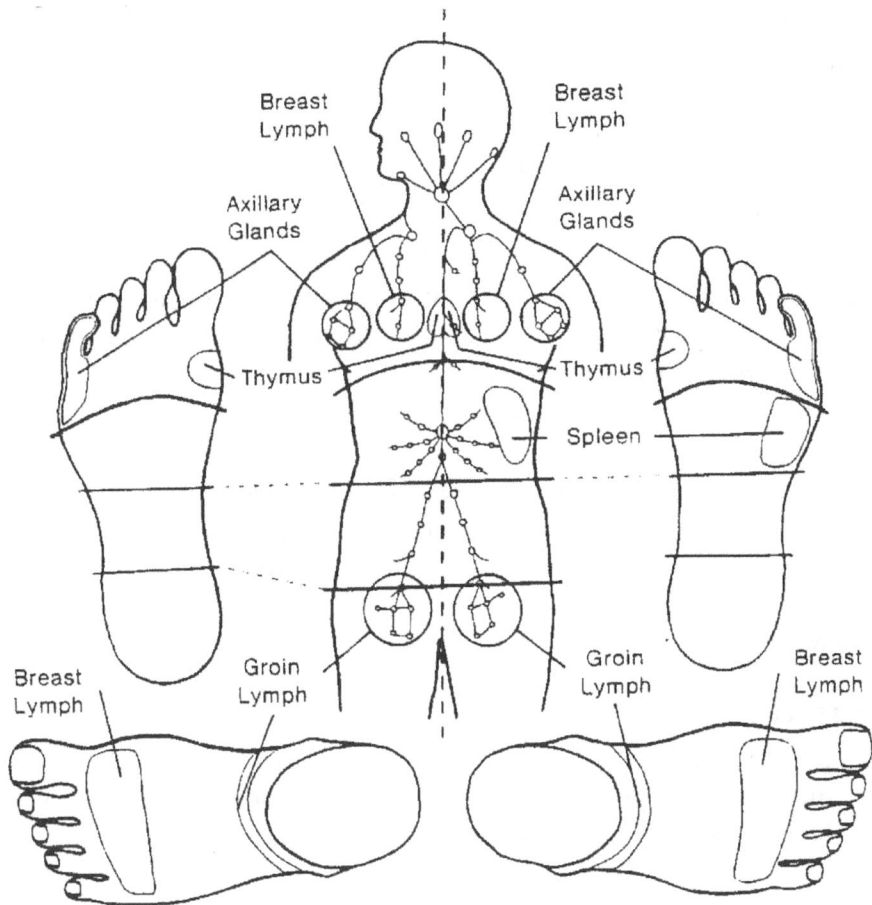

The Lymphatic system, which acts not only as part of the immune system but also as a purifying or drainage system for the body, when it is put under strain because of injury or unhealthy life styles. Waste products cannot be filtered out quickly enough and build up, causing swelling in and around the Lymph Nodes.

Lymph drainage is a gentle, pumping massage which aims to speed up the removal of waste products by stimulating the lymphatic system. The technique is very useful on anyone with swelling or any injury, particularly a sports injury. Fluid retention may be relieved, and even acne and eczema as wellas other related disorders may improve.

All the movements are performed up the body towards the nearest lymph nodes, starting nearest the centre of the body and moving out to the extremities. Since lymph vessels are close to the surface, your pressure should be very light. It is hard to believe that something so gentle could be so effective, but the following massage will demonstrate the success of such a light massage on a swollen ankle.

Few things are more relaxing than a good foot massage, tired feet suddenly feel light again and the whole body is refreshed. The foot, particularly the sole, contains thousands of nerve endings, and by massaging these you can stimulate not only the feet but also the whole body. Regular foot massage helps to keep the feet flexible and healthy.

To begin, work on only one foot at a time, you need use only a little oil to work with because more will make you slip and slide too much. Start by stroking the feet from the toes toward the body, this will help the client to become accustomed to your touch and also help them to relax.

When you reach the ankle swing your hands around and return to the toes with a lighter stroke. Thisis a warming movement that will gently increase the temperature of the feet (a good move for clients with cold feet).

Foot Lymphatic Massage

THUMB STROKING

> Support the foot with your fingers underneath it and place your thumbs on top at the base of the toes. Stroke up the foot with your thumbs, in a fanning motion, out to the sides and gliding backto the toes.

> Next stroke with your thumbs working alternately. Stroke up with one thumb as the other glides back down the side. The movement can be a little longer than before, reaching up to the ankle.

TOE MASSAGE

> Loosen and warm the whole area by wriggling the toes. Sandwich the foot just above the toes and rotate your hands in a bicycle peddling motion. Massage each toe individually, Squeeze gently and rotate each toe with a gentle twisting or pulling action towards you.

> To finish, clasp all the toes with one hand and bend them backwards and forwards to encourage flexibility.

TENDON STROKING

Support the foot with both hands, with your fingers underneath and your thumbs on top. Stoke in each furrow between the toes covering the tendons, one thumb following the other. Run your thumbs up the foot towards the ankle, doing about four strokes in each furrow.

Another method is, to make a fist with one hand and place the knuckles on the sole of the foot.Push the thumb of the other hand into the fist of the first hand and using your index finger,caterpillar along the tendons between the toes for as far as you can reach.

PRESSURES

Support the foot with your fingers on top and your thumbs underneath. Press firmly on the solewith one thumb on top of the other for three to seven seconds, then move on about half an inchand repeat. Work all over the ball of the foot and in a line down the centre to the heel. Then do more pressures in lines on either side of this central line.

STROKING THE ARCH

Sooth the foot by stroking the arch, rest one hand on top of the foot and stroke firmly into the main arch, using the heel of your other hand. Curve your hand back to fit the shape of the foot,and stroke from the ball of the foot to the heel. return with a light stroke to start again. Repeat at least four times.

KNUCKLING

Keep one hand on top of the foot and curl the fingers of the other hand to make a loose fist sothat you can massage the foot with the middle section of your fingers. Move your fingers round to make rippling rotary movements. work firmly all over the sole. Draw steadily down over the sole of the foot from the toes to the heel to create a deep satisfying stretch. This will help keep the feet supple and flexible.

ROTARY PRESSURES

Stroke the whole foot as you did to warm up, then apply circular pressures all round the ankle with one hand on each side. Press firmly on the upwards sweep of the circle, as you move towards the leg, and keep the pressure light on the return. Use your middle fingers on the sides and back of the ankle, then your thumbs on the front.

SPECIALISED LYMPH DRAINAGE

With the legs extended, place four fingers of each hand on either side of the ankles and using spiral movement in a clockwise direction move upwards on each side of the Achilles tendon toterminate around the mid calf area.

Follow by using alternating thumb circles lightly over the ankle bones, and over the Dorsal aspect with alternating thumb fanning movements. Apply pressure over the Transverse Arch from the outside towards the centre with circular upward movements. Finish by gentle stroking movements up the lower leg from shin to calf.

When looking at the feet from a therapist standpoint, the patients right foot represents thepatients right side of the body and the patients left foot represents the patients left side. The diaphragm is in proportion to the discolouration border on the sole of the feet. The waist line corresponds to the waist of the patient and the heel line is in proportion to the discolouration border on the heel of the foot.

MERIDIANS OF THE LOWER EXTREMITY

These diagrams are for interest only, they are not part of the reflexology experience, but they are connected to the modality.

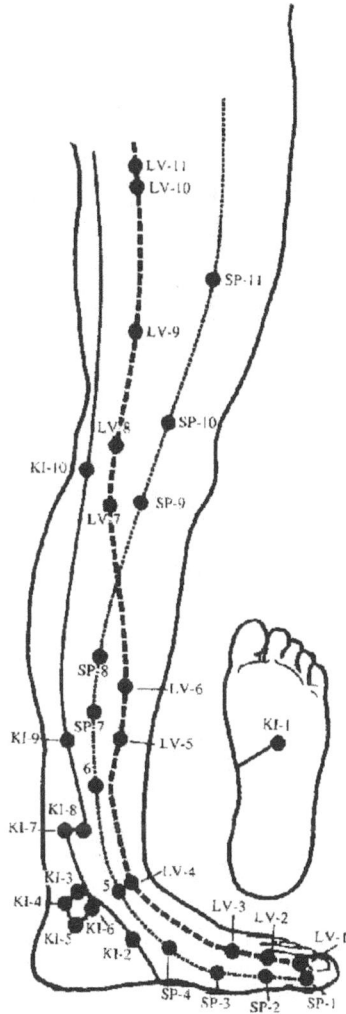

Kidney, Spleen and Liver meridians are found on the inner (medial) leg. These are Yin organs.

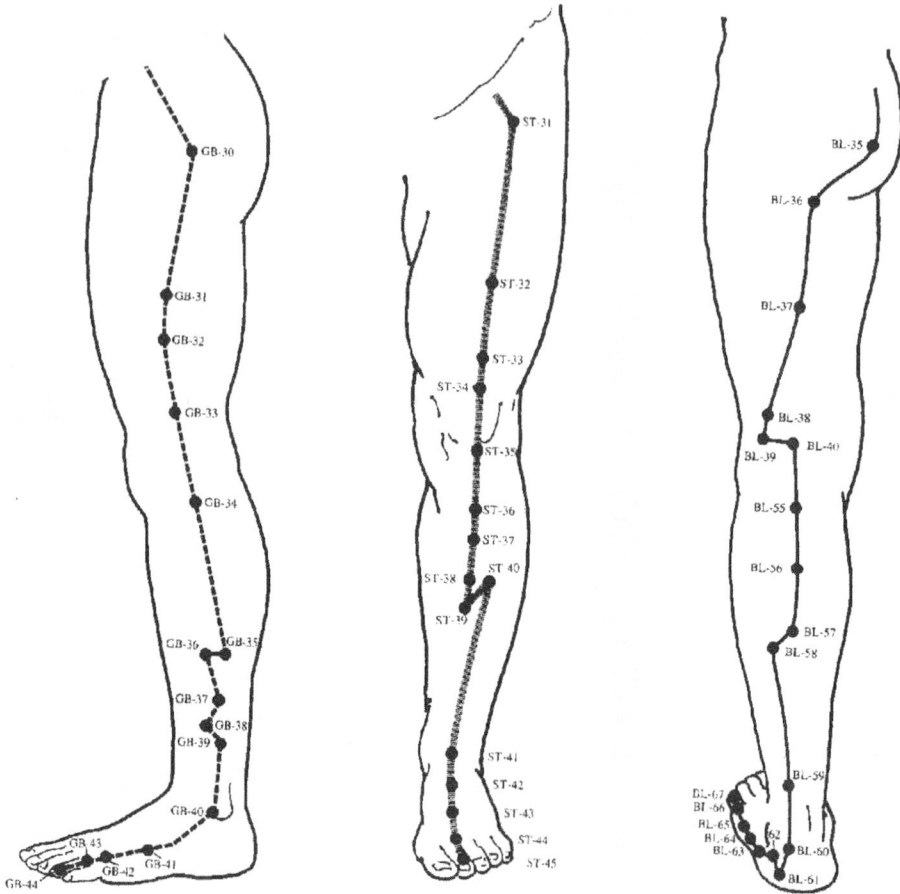

Urinary Bladder, Gall Bladder, and Stomach Channels are found on the outer (lateral) leg.

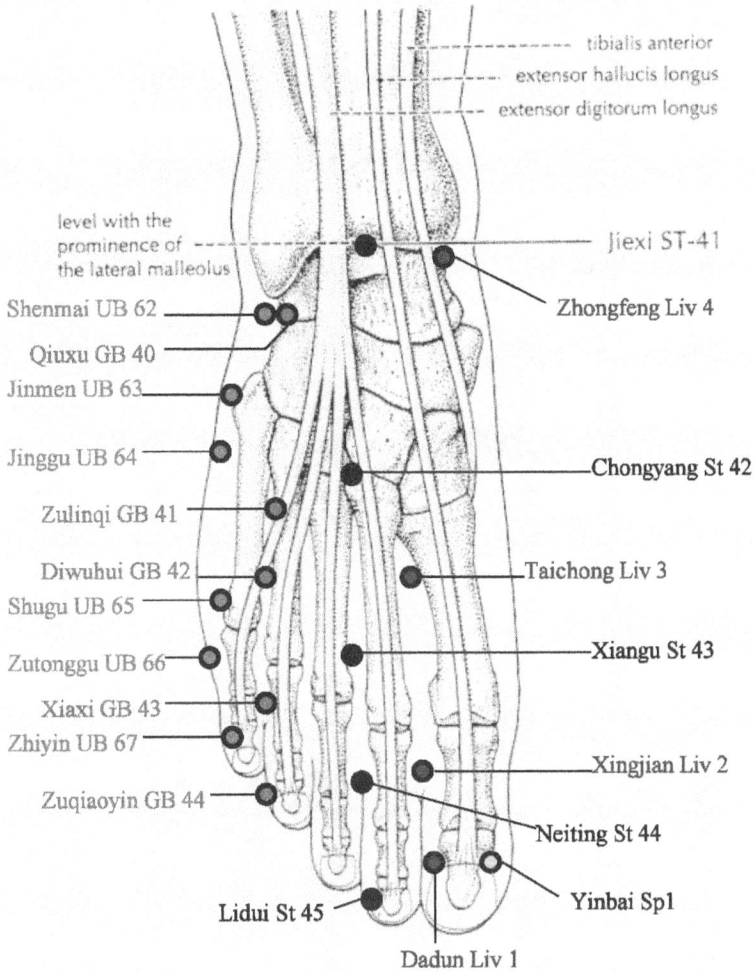

tibialis anterior
extensor hallucis longus
extensor digitorum longus

level with the
prominence of
the lateral malleolus

Jiexi ST-41

Shenmai UB 62

Zhongfeng Liv 4

Qiuxu GB 40

Jinmen UB 63

Jinggu UB 64

Chongyang St 42

Zulinqi GB 41

Diwuhui GB 42

Taichong Liv 3

Shugu UB 65

Xiangu St 43

Zutonggu UB 66

Xiaxi GB 43

Zhiyin UB 67

Xingjian Liv 2

Zuqiaoyin GB 44

Neiting St 44

Yinbai Sp1

Lidui St 45

Dadun Liv 1

If you were to put extra energy into the following areas, you might be surprised as to the results. I have high-lighted the following points and given a few suggestions as to how they can help. Try using circular finger or thumb pressure on these points to assist your treatment protocol.

Putting emphasis on the following Acu-Pressure points will help with the following problems:

UB 62	Headaches, pain, fevers, depression	GB 40	Chest pain, breathing difficulties
UB 63	Cramps, Knee pain, back pain	GB 41	Pain and tight chest, headaches
UB 64	Relaxes the muscles & alleviates pain	GB 42	headaches, itchy eyes, tinitus

39

UB 65	Clears head, reduces swelling, pain	GB 43	Headaches, Chest pain, Knee pain
UB 66	Neck pain, fever, vomiting	GB 44	Nightmares, sweaty hands and feet
UB 67	Headaches, ear problems, chest pain	St 41	Ankle swelling, abdominal distention
St 42	Swollen foot, manic-depressive	Liv 1	Urinary & menstrual problems
St 43	Swollen foot, abdominal pain	Liv 2	Eye disorders, Chest & knee pain
St 44	Swollen foot, Cold hands and feet	Liv 3	Heart problems, insomnia
St 45	Cold limbs, swollen knees	Liv 4	low grade fever, knee & foot pain

Medial aspect

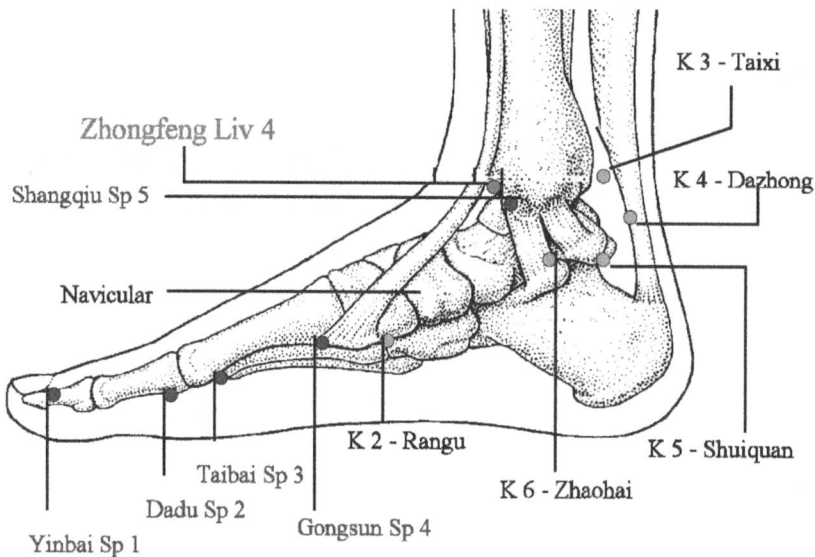

Sp 1	Swollen limbs, diarrhea, cold feet	K 1	Insomnia, coughing, constipation
Sp 2	Abdominal distention, insomnia	K 2	Sore throat, night sweats, infertility
Sp 3	Abdominal pain, knee and thigh pain	K 3	Ear problems, Coughs, heart problems

Sp 4	Stomach pain, pain in heel & sole of feet	K 4	Constipation, Swollen heel, sore throat
Sp 5	Ankle & inner thigh pain	K 5	Menstrual & urinary problems

Underlying Causes of Illness

TOXICITY

The underlying causes of illness are:

- pH imbalances
- Too many toxins
- Bowel imbalances
- Adrenal exhaustion
- Cellular distress
- Emotional distress
- Too little oxygen

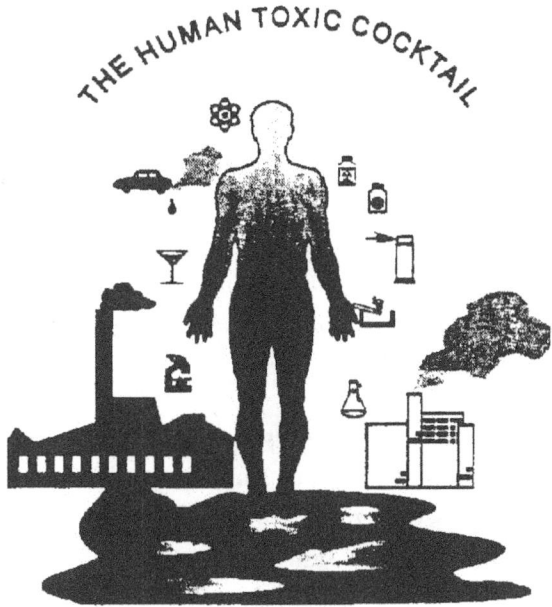

THE HUMAN TOXIC COCKTAIL

Physicians are seeing an increase in "Non-Specific Symptoms" like chronic fatigue, migraines, headaches, SARS, sinus congestion etc. People just don't "feel good" anymore. They become more susceptible to colds or "bugs". Autoimmune diseases like arthritis and MS etc. are on the rise.

Avoiding food additives and drinking purified water are no longer sufficient because we are being exposed to toxins at home, work and recreational areas throughout the day and night. The body has a certain capacity to detox itself, but when this is exceeded it builds-up around the cells causing a wide variety of problems.

Conventional medicine will not help, laboratory testing will not indicate the presence of toxins in the body, but symptoms will persist, occurring rarely, sporadically, frequently or on a daily basis. Ignoring them or failing to detoxify the body can eventually lead to chronic system toxicity which results in damage to internal organs, tissues and systems.

Once a detox program begins the recipient often feels rapid relief from chronic complaints and start to feel better within a few weeks. Everyone has a different level of toxic load tolerance, and an individual ability to deal with it. When you reach that level you're in overload, from there its downhill.

Your tolerance and susceptibility can be influenced by:
- Your overall health
- Your emotional state
- Inherited, constitutional or genetic weaknesses
- Stressors
- Environment

Some of the most common symptoms are:

Fatigue, drowsiness, headaches, migraine, restlessness, irritability, rashes, nausea, joint aches, tinitis, swollen glands, hormonal imbalances, hair loss, difficulty concentrating, dizziness, oedema, lethargy, system degeneration....

Note: these symptoms can also occur in disorders that are not related to toxins, which is why diagnostic biological testing are necessary to trace the cause and to determine the optimal treatment.

Four Steps to Wellness

Through Education and understanding
1. reduce your susceptibility to toxins;
2. detox the body;
3. clean up your home, work and recreational environment; and
4. reduce or prevent future exposure.

The Physiological Perspective

Over 90% of the body is fluid.
60% of the body is toxic already (germs and bacteria)

Extracellular fluid bathes the external surfaces of cells, contained within the fluid you will find, dissolved minerals, nutrients, metabolic waste etc. This fluid is in constant motion and as a part of its ionic nature these fluids form a communication network carrying information throughout the body. It moves between the bloodstream and the tissues delivering nutrients, and removing waste products. So you can see, if these pathways become clogged or congested, a traffic-jam can result in a rapid build-up of waste products causing deposits to be laid-down that will add to the problem. (Like a river overflowing its banks and depositing silt and soil in the town) as well as starvation of needed nutrients to the cells and tissues. Age also causes a slowing down of the exchange especially within the systems (veins, lymph).

Everything we eat, drink and inhale or touch enters our body and must be broken-down or eliminated to avoid depositing phase into tissues and cells, if the fluid that bathes the cells and tissues is toxic, the metabolic by-products will accumulate. Such toxins as heavy metals, agricultural chemicals and air or water pollution may deposit in the fatty tissues, liver, kidney, reproductive organs or nervous system.

For example, lead poisoning causes brain damage, ozone irritates lungs, pesticides cause liver/kidney damage etc.

Mental/Emotional Toxins
- Disease forming belief systems
- Traumas (emotional/physical)
- A negative subconscious
- Learned negative patterns

Inherited Toxins
- Inherited from the mothers blood, genetic DNA

Physical Toxins
- Metabolic waste (Uric acid, Metabolic by-products, Urea, Lactic acid)
- Free radical damage
- Digestive waste (Dysbiosis, incomplete digestion)
- Natural environmental pollutants (Radon, heavy metals, pollens, plants,)
- Man-made pollutants (Chemicals, pesticides, preservatives, industry, radiation)

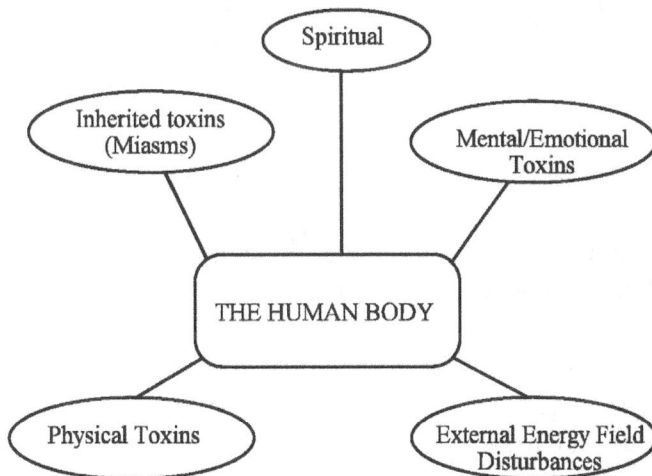

Spiritual

Inherited toxins
(Miasms)

Mental/Emotional
Toxins

THE HUMAN BODY

Physical Toxins

External Energy Field
Disturbances

Biological organisms and their by-products:	Viruses, Bacteria, Parasites and funguses
Residues of medicinal and recreational drugs:	Marijuana, steroids and opiates

External Energy Field Disturbances:
- Geopathic stress, (earths magnetic field).
- Electromagnetic, (high voltage cables, in-home electrical cables, computers/TV's etc.)
- Radiation (X-rays, Nuclear, ultraviolet etc.)
- Frequency disturbances (colour, sound, radio, etc.)

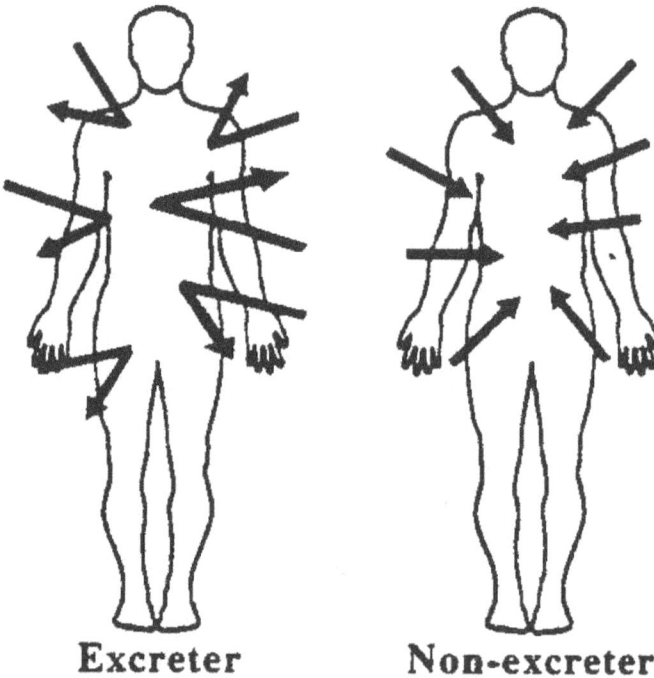

Excreter   **Non-excreter**

We need to be excreters not non-excreters. As long as we retain toxins we will be harbouring sickness that will manifest one way or another as time goes by.

Bowel sluggishness contributes the most towards bowel toxicity than anything else. By stimulating the Large Intestine area you will be contributing to less toxins in the body and so contribute to better health long term.

TOXIC BIO-ACCUMULATION & HEALTH

Health related effects of toxic residue bio-accumulation and environmental stresses:

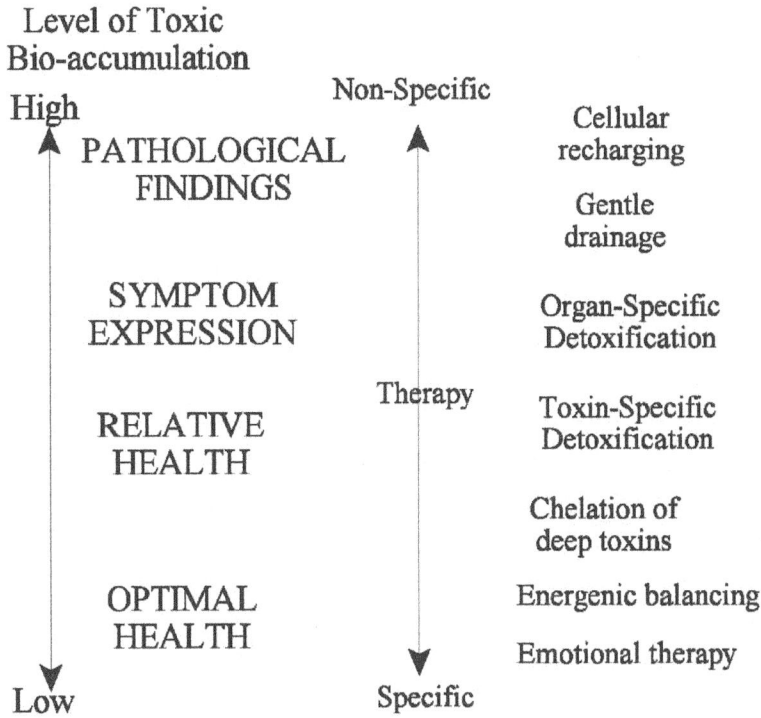

Level of Toxic
Bio-accumulation

High

Non-Specific

PATHOLOGICAL
FINDINGS

Cellular
recharging

Gentle
drainage

SYMPTOM
EXPRESSION

Organ-Specific
Detoxification

Therapy

RELATIVE
HEALTH

Toxin-Specific
Detoxification

Chelation of
deep toxins

OPTIMAL
HEALTH

Energenic balancing

Emotional therapy

Low

Specific

BIO-ENERGETIC TOXICOLOGY

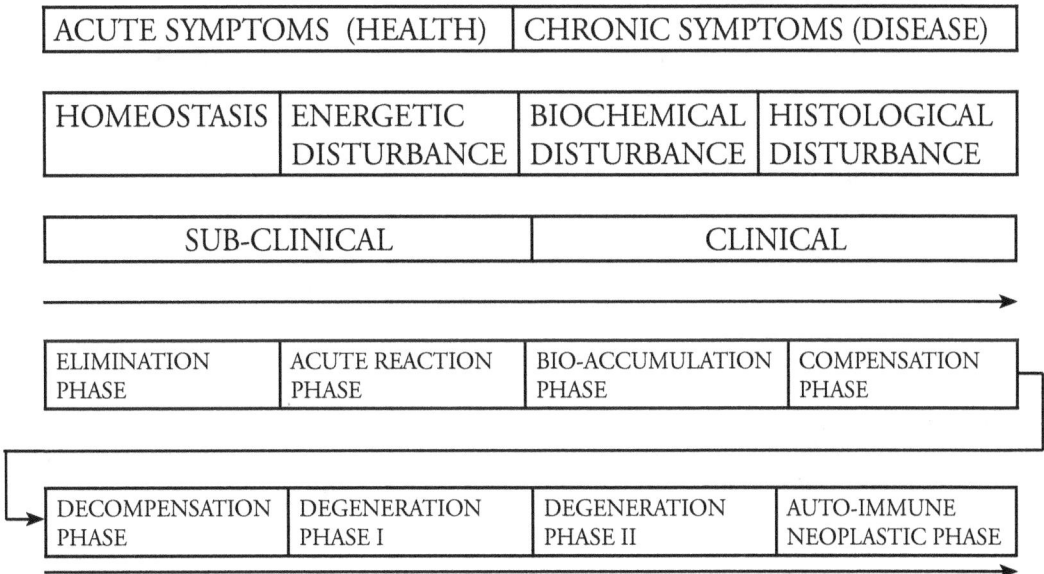

ACUTE SYMPTOMS (HEALTH)	CHRONIC SYMPTOMS (DISEASE)		

HOMEOSTASIS	ENERGETIC DISTURBANCE	BIOCHEMICAL DISTURBANCE	HISTOLOGICAL DISTURBANCE

SUB-CLINICAL	CLINICAL

ELIMINATION PHASE	ACUTE REACTION PHASE	BIO-ACCUMULATION PHASE	COMPENSATION PHASE

DECOMPENSATION PHASE	DEGENERATION PHASE I	DEGENERATION PHASE II	AUTO-IMMUNE NEOPLASTIC PHASE

47

Elimination Phase

The body will normally neutralize toxins in the organs and tissues and eliminate them via faeces, urine, sweat, menstrual flow and discharge from nose, ears, wounds.

Acute Reaction Phase

When the body does not succeed in removing all toxins by normal elimination, it will try to remove them by acute reactions such as, fever, vomiting, diarrhea, inflammation and skin eruptions.

Bio-accumulation Phase

This is where the bodies elimination processes fail to remove toxins and will lead to chronic cellular stress, benign tumors, gout, liver, kidney and pancreas irritation.

Compensation Phase

This phase begins after toxins have been laid-down and the body adapts to the increase by discontinuing the symptoms. But, is the pre-degeneration phase or what we call pre-cancerous condition.

De-compensation Phase

This is where the body can no longer compensate for the toxicity, it will begin to deteriorate physically. Acute symptoms reappear like, acne, fatigue, headaches, inflammation, PMS, allergiesand susceptibility to infections.

Degeneration Phase I

This phase is the beginning of biochemical and histological changes indicative of cell damage, appearing as arthritis, emphysema, premature aging, memory loss etc.

Degeneration Phase II

This is characterized by emotional and physical changes as the body reacts to degeneration.Symptoms become unbearable, a time when symptomatic suppression medication is used the most, depression and despair are common at this point.

Auto-immune Neoplastic Phase

The malignant stage, auto-immune reactions develop, life threatening disease is present. Death is not far away.....

WHAT'S THE SOLUTION...
detox

The Detox Process
The majority of detoxification is carried out by the four systems:

1. Respiratory
2. Digestive
3. Urinary
4. Dermal

Foot Disorders

SKIN CARE

Our skin expresses the physical tension of our bodies, and as such the skin will reflect the overall health of the person. Reflexology relaxes the entire body as well as the mind and spirit. Once this tension is released the body can begin to rejuvenate itself more readily.

Apart from the basic information and historical evidence contained in this course, which I hope will stimulate your appetite to know more and to become part of the growing awareness in the field of complementary health care, in particular, Reflexology. I sincerely hope that those of you who will go on to become Reflexologists will experience both the joy of learning and the interest in treating the people who turn to Reflexologists for help, often after they have exhausted every other form of conventional therapy as well as complimentary healthcare. The most incredible fact about illness is that it can happen to any one of us, no matter what our colour, race or creed. I have successfully treated people from all walks of life, they have come to me in their chauffeur-driven cars and others have had to walk or taken a bus. They have paid me with cash, or I have even accepted on many occasions payment in the form of a bag of produce grown in their own gardens because they were short of money.

I always say to my students that they must not turn people away just because they are unable to find sufficient funds for a treatment. There are certain qualities that make a good Reflexologist other than qualifications. I can honestly say that I have never once in my rewarding career ever felt bored,or not looked upon each day as one that would bring me in touch with more people who I am more than pleased to meet and help.

FOOT DISEASES/DISORDERS

Verruca -Warts

Warts are contagious growths, caused by a virus. They are very common in childhood as well as the teen years. The prevalence of them tend to decline in adulthood, due to the body building up a resistance to the virus. However, warts are more difficult to get rid of in adults, than at any other age.

There are over 50 types of wart viruses (ie; finger warts, genital warts, planters warts). There are various methods of wart removal. Some involve a frequent application of topical acids that slowly eat away at the virus. This is done in conjunction with a paring down of the callus. The drawback to this method is the length of the treatment.

Warts tend to be like weeds, very deep and stubborn to get rid of. Faster methods include cryotherapy, (liquid nitrogen freezing). The nitrogen at 196 degrees C, is applied or sprayed on the wart. A carbon dioxide laser is another option available. All of these methods involve some form of painful residue, specifically if the warts are found on the fingertips or feet. These are areas of heightened tactile sensation. The holistic method of treating warts is through the use of a high quality lemon essential oil. The oil is applied directly over the needed area 4- 6 times daily. It is painless and extremely effective. Also Infra-Red or Laser light is often very effective as well.

Club Foot (talipes equinovarus)

This can be a hereditary malformation of the foot and ankle bones, sometimes resulting from intrauterine (pertaining to the inside of the uterus) constriction (muscle spasm) during childbirth and characterized by unilateral (involving only one side) or bilateral (involving both sides) deviation of the metatarsal bones of the forefoot. Generally the heel turns in and under the ankle, the inner edge of the foot turns up and the front of one foot turns in toward the other. The entire sole of the foot and toes flex downwards.

Treatment: Treatment depends on the extent and rigidity of the deformity. Splints and casts in infancy may produce correction, surgery may be used in more profound cases to assist normal function. Aesthetics care is needed to help nail growth and skin and lymph care, as the foot shape causes nail and pressure areas that will need to be addressed.

Flatfoot (Pes Planus or Pes Planovalgus)

Pronation, flatfoot, and pes Planovalgus are recognized by flattened medial longitudinal arch with outward rolling of the foot. This foot condition may be caused by loose ligaments in the foot which are unable to hold the bones in position, resulting in the rear of the heel and the front of the foot abnormally turned outward. This repositioning flattens the arch of the foot, hence "flatfoot".

Treatment: There is none, but good foot hygiene is important as pressure points occur in this condition much easier than in a well developed foot.

Bunion (hallux valgus deformity)

This is an abnormal enlargement of the joint at the base of the great toe. Normally caused by inflammation of the bursa, usually as a result of chronic irritation and pressure from poorly fittedshoes.

People with bunions usually have traumatic subluxations (a partial abnormal separation of the articular surfaces of a joint) and pain in the second metatarsophalangeal articulations (joints). Painful subluxation of the metatarsophalangeal (pertaining to the metatarsal bones of the foot) articulation also can be caused by arthropathies (any disease or abnormal condition effecting a joint) such as Rheumatoid arthritis.

A deviation in the big toe joint caused by stretched tendons placing enormous tension on the bigtoe. This tension eventually forces the toe to deviate to the outside with the top of the toe pointingtowards the baby toe.

Treatment: Anti-inflammatory drugs, or Essential oils. Rest and elevate the effected limb. Increase lymph drainage to help remove swelling and inflammation.

Chilblain

Chilblains are due to an injury by cold causing structural and functional disturbances of small blood vessels, cells, nerve and skin. A skin condition resulting in itching, burning, blistering and ulceration that are similar to a thermal burn, may occur. The skin may become red and swollen generally this condition is caused by exposure to cold or cold water.

Treatment: Protection from further exposure to cold, gentle warming. Later a medicinal skin care preparation may be tolerated by the skin to hasten the healing process, or an Aromatherapy skin-care preparation could be prepared by a qualified Aromatherapists and applied directly to the skin without delay.

Athletes Foot (Tinea Pedis)

This is a contagious fungal infection usually starting in between the 3rd and 4th inter-digital (between the toes) spaces and later involve the plantar surface (sole) of the arch. The infected area has a reddish line around it, while inside is a whitish flaking of the skin where the fungus is growing. It has the appearance of onion-skin peeling (the bodies attempt at ridding itself of the fungus). There may be a burning or an itching sensation present. Infected toenails become thickened and distorted. Always keep feet dry and dry well in between toes. Fungal infections thrive in a damp, moist environment.

Wear natural fibre socks and use an anti-fungal medication at the first instance of athletes foot.

Treatment: Drying the feet well after bathing and applying powder between the toes will help prevent it. Essential Oil of Ti-Tree is very effective and the Allopathic medical treatment would be:
"Griseofulvin" or "Miconazole" and "Tolnaftate".

Griseofulvin: An Anti-fungal drug given by mouth when creams and lotions fail to eliminate the problem.

Miconazole: An Anti-fungal cream or lotion.

Tolnaftate: Available over the counter as an Anti-fungal cream, powder, liquid, aerosol powder and aerosol liquid.

Plantar Warts
A viral infection named after their location. (plantar = bottom of the foot) They may appear on the heel or the ball of the foot. Plantar warts are similar in appearance to a callus, but a wart will have tiny black dots in them, these black dots that are characteristic of a wart are the tiny blood vessels that are nourishing it. Often flattened by pressure and surrounded by carnified epithelium. The virus that causes these warts must enter through an abrasion or a puncture wound, once the virus enters, the wart spreads and multiplies to form a painful growth. It is generally painful due to the location of them on the weight-bearing part of the foot. They may be exquisitely tender and can be distinguished from corns and calluses by their tendency to pinpoint bleeding when the surface is pared away. Mosaic warts are plaques of myriad small, closely set plantar warts. By trimming away the horny layer of a plantar wart it will appear sharply circumscribed, sometimes with a soft macerated tissue or with central black dots resulting from thrombosed capillaries, and paring it will cause pinpoint bleeding.

Treatment: Aromatherapy would use Essential Oil of Lemon 4-6 times a day, one drop of oil directly onto the effected area. A Doctor may apply or treat with "Salicylic Acid, Cantharidin, Electrodesiccation, Solid Carbon Dioxide, or Liquid Nitrogen".

Callus
A superficial circumscribed area of hyper-keratosis at a site of repeated trauma, where a build up of thick skin occurs, serving as a protective barrier. It is generally

caused by pressure and friction on the affected area. They are commonly found on the heel and the ball of the foot as well as at the sideof the big toe and the bunion area. The hands are also afflicted with this problem. Trimming away a callus means the removal of the heaped-up keratin, the skin markings (fingerprint type lines) are preserved.

Treatment: Trimming away a callus carefully using a bladed instrument or using a rough stone or sand paper abrasive.

Corns

A painful conical hyper-keratosis, found principally over toe joints and between toes. A protrusion on the top or the side of the toe produced in response to the contraction of the offending toe or from improperly fitted footwear.

Corns are pea-sized or slightly larger, they ache spontaneously and may be tender to pressure. By trimming away the horny layer of a corn, shows a sharply outlined translucent core that interrupts the normal papillary line.

Treatment: Trimming away a corn carefully using a bladed instrument or using a rough stone or sand paper abrasive. You can temporarily relieve corn pain by using a doughnut-shaped corn pad, this will take the pressure off the corn. The two types of corn-pads available are; none-medicated and medicated. The medicated pads contain an acid to help dissolve the corn, their drawback is they tend to cause infection if not cleaned and looked after properly. People with Diabetes or circulation problems should not use them because the skin is too sensitive to the acids.

Hammer Toe

A toe that is contracted/bent and permanently flexed at the mid-phalangeal joint, possibly causingpain and resulting in a clawlike appearance. Because of the position of the hammer toe, more often than not there will be a corn present as well. Hammer toes may be caused from poor fitting footwear.

Treatment: Provide support, wear sandals, buy well fitting custom-made shoes. As a last resort consider surgery to correct the problem. The most important method is prevention.

NAIL DISEASES/DISORDERS

Fungal Nails

Also known as onychomycosis. The fungus gives the nail a discolouration. (yellowish) and the nail is generally detached from the nail bed in the affected area. This is not a painful condition. It is just unpleasant to look at.

Treatment: Apply Essential Oils of Ti-tree directly onto the effected nails also Vick's vapour rub seems to work well also.

Ingrown Toenails

This occurs when a toenail becomes embedded in the surrounding skin of the toe. The upper corner(s) of the toenail grows into the skin surrounding the nail. It becomes increasingly tender and an infection may develop. It can be caused by improper cutting of the toenails. Best solution is to pack the toenail to help relieve the pressure.

Treatment: Soak the feet in warm water with Epsom Salts for 15 minutes to soften the nail andsurrounding skin. Gently pull the skin away from the trapped nail. After the nail and the skin has been separated you can plug a small piece of cotton between the nail and the skin for a few days untilthe nail grows out and the skin heals. Carefully trimming the nail with a pair of toe nail clippers is another way to keep it from burrowing further into the skin, but this method is not recommended.

To avoid a recurrence of ingrown toenails, it helps to trim your nails properly. When cutting be sureto cut straight across, and round off the edges slightly with a nail file. There are many disorders that can be manicured. These conditions are basically nail irregularities. Any client having any infection or irritation present should be referred to a physician. Corrugations or wavy ridges are caused by an uneven growth of the nails, usually the result of illness or injury.

Furrows (depressions)

These can run either lengthwise or across the nail. These are usually the result of illness or an injury to the nail cells in or near the matrix. They can also be caused by pregnancy or stress. These nails may be fragile, and if so, manicure with care.

Leuconychia (white spots)

These appear frequently in the nails. They are caused by injury to the base of the nail. as the nailgrows, the white spots will eventually disappear.

Onychauxis (or hypertrophy)
This is an overgrowth of the nail in thickness. It is usually caused by a local infection and can also be hereditary. Do not manicure the nail if the infection is present.

Onychatrophia (or atrophy of the nail)
This causes the nail to lose its lustre, become smaller, and sometimes shed entirely. This may becaused by either injury or disease.

Pterygium
This is the forward growth of the cuticle that adheres to the base of the nail. It can be caused by circulatory problems. Gently nip off any excess cuticle with nippers.

Onychorrhexis
This is the condition of split of brittle nails. It could be caused by an injury to the finger, impropernail filing, vitamin deficiencies, illness or excessive chemical use (ie; harsh alkalies, polish removers etc.)

Hangnail
This is a condition in which the cuticle splits around the nail. They may be caused by dryness, cutting off too much cuticle, or improper removal.

Eggshell Nails
These are nails that have a noticeably thin, white nail plate and are more flexible than normal. The nail plate separates from the nail bed and curves at the free edge. It can be caused by a chronic illness of systemic origin or nervous origin.

Blue Nails
These can be caused by poor blood circulation or a heart disorder. The client may still receive a normal manicure.

Bruised Nails
These will have a dark purplish, black or brown spot that is generally due to injury and bleeding inthe nail bed. The dried blood attaches itself to the nail and grows out with it.

Nail Diseases
There are a number of nail diseases that may be encountered during manicures. Any nail disease should be referred to a physician. Do not manicure any nail that shows a sign of infection .

Onychosis
This is a technical term applied to a nail disease.

Onychomycosis (tinea ungium, or ringworm of the nails)
This is an infectious disease caused by a fungus. A common form is whitish patches that can be scraped off the surface. A second form is long, yellowish streaks within the nail. The disease invades the free edge and spreads towards the root. The infected portion is thick and discoloured. In the third form, the deeper layers of the nail are infected, causing superficial layers to appear irregularly thin. The infected layers peel off and expose the diseased parts of the nail bed.

Ringworm of the foot (athletes foot)
In acute conditions, deep itchy, colourless vesicles appear. They appear singly, in groups, and sometimes on only one foot. They spread over the sole and between the toes, perhaps involving the nail fold and infecting the nail. When the vesicles rupture, the skin becomes red and oozes. The lesions dry as they heal. Fungal infections of the feet are likely to become chronic. Both the prevention of the infection and the beneficial treatment are accomplished by keeping the skin cool, dry and clean.

Paronychia (or felon)
This is an infectious and inflammatory condition of the tissues surrounding the nails. It is alsocharacterized by gradual thickening of the nail plate. This condition is caused by a bacterial infection.

Onychia
This is an inflammation of the nail matrix, accompanied by pus formation. Improperly sanitized nailimplements and bacterial infection can cause this disease.

Onychoptosis
This is the periodic shedding of one or more nails, either in part or in whole. This condition might follow certain diseases such as syphilis.

Onycholysis
This is a loosening of the nail, without shedding. It is frequently associated with an internal disorder.

Onychopyma
This denotes a swelling of the nail.

Onyschophosis
This refers to a growth of horny epithelium in the nail bed.

Onychogryposis
This pertains to enlarged and increased curvature of the nails.

The History of Reflexology

HISTORY AND ORIGINS OF REFLEXOLOGY

Reflexology is a method for activating the inner healing powers of the body. It is both old, and new. From different ancient texts, we have found illustrations, and artifacts relating to the art of reflexology. We know that the early Chinese, Japanese, Indian, Russian and Egyptians worked on the feet to promote good health. Today many of these same techniques have been developed into a modern scientific method which we call Reflexology. What joins the ancients with the moderns is the long-established principle that there are energy zones that run throughout the body and reflex areas in the feet that correspond to all the major organs, glands, and body parts.

Dr. William Fitzgerald

At the beginning of the twentieth century Dr. William Fitzgerald, an American medical doctor, developed the modern zone theory of the human body, arguing that parts of the body have corresponding areas to parts of the feet. Dr. Edwin Bowers, Fitzgerald's colleague, used a dramatic demonstration to convince others of the theory's validity. He showed that he could stick a pin into a volunteer's face without causing pain if he first applied pressure to the point in the person's hand which corresponded to that area of the face.

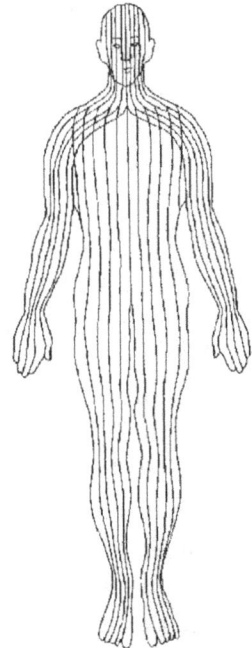

Eunice Ingham

In the 1930s, Eunice Ingham, a physiotherapist for Dr. Joseph Shelby Riley,who was also a student and advocate of reflexology, used zone therapy in her work with patients. She concluded that, since the zones ran throughout the body and could be accessed anywhere, some areas might

Zone Therapy

be more accessible and effective than others. She was right. The feet were the most responsive areas for working the zones because they were extremely sensitive. Eventually, she mapped the entire body onto the feet and discovered that an alternating pressure on the various points had therapeutic effects far beyond the limits of just reducing pain, to which zone therapy had been previously employed. And so Reflexology was born.

Modern Reflexology is both a science and an art. As a science, it requires careful study, faithfulpractice, a sound knowledge of the techniques, and skill. And yet as one of the healing arts, Reflexology yields the best results when the reflexologist works with dedication, patience, focussed attention and above all, loving care.

What Is Reflexology

Reflexology is a form of "holistic healing", the term "holistic" being taken from the Greek word"holos", meaning "whole". In accordance with any holistic principle, three aspects must be invoked in order to achieve a feeling of well-being. These are a balanced mind, body and spirit. Reflexology is taught in three different forms, body, hand and foot Reflexology. The latter is the most popular form of treatment as the feet not only get more abuse than the rest of our body, but also because it is more responsive and sensitive to external stimulus than the hands.

Hand Reflexology is helpful for treatments that are not accessible in the feet, for instance, when the feet are injured or too sensitive for positive treatment to be given. Body Reflexology is more in line with Acupressure point stimulation of the meridian lines. To answer the question at the beginning in brief, You could describe Reflexology as treating the feet by applying pressure to different parts of the feet to stimulate the various organs associated with these reflex areas.

Where Did it Originate

Reflexology has a recorded history of use for over 5000 years in Egypt, India and China. In the year 1027 A.D., it was used in China for energy-balancing. Dr Wang Wei in ancient China had a human figure cast in bronze. On this bronze figure he marked those points on the body that he believed were important for acupuncture. The students practised on this bronze figure, locating acupuncture points, which eventually helped them to find those same points on the human body. When this knowledge was put into practice in treating the sick, practitioners positioned the needles in the appropriate areas of the body and then applied deep pressure therapy on the soles, inside, and outside edge of both feet, they then applied a concentrated pressure on the big toe. The reason they used the feet in conjunction with the acupuncture needles was to channel extra energy through the body. Dr. Wang Wei said that the feet were the most sensitive part of all and contained great energizing areas.

EGYPTIAN REFLEXOLOGY TREATMENT
Copied from the tomb of Ankhmahor around 2330 B.C.

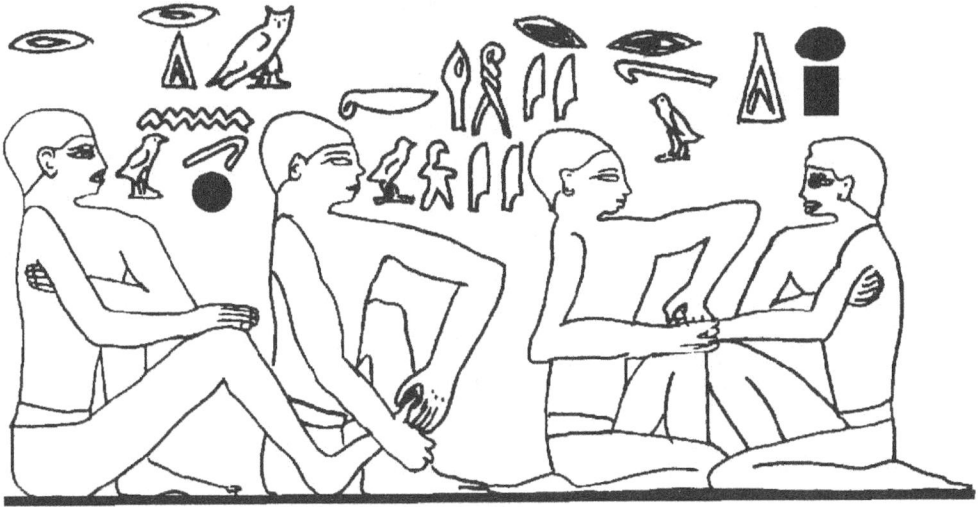

In 1916 Dr. Edwin Bowers described the treatment developed by Dr Fitzgerald, as "zone therapy". One year later their combined work appeared in the book "Zone therapy", which contained medical recommendations for doctors, dentists, gynaecologists, chiropractors, and ear, nose and throats pecialists. During the past twenty years reflexology has been making a slow but steady impact in the field of complementary health care therapies. Possibly because it has proved to be one of the few safe and effective ways of stimulating the functions of organs and other parts of the body, withoutthe need for drugs.

Before we look at how and why reflexology works, lets consider its many benefits.

BENEFITS

Stress cannot be avoided. We live with it and in it everyday. In itself, stress is neither good nor bad.Playing tennis or giving a dinner party is stressful and yet exhilarating and fun. Stress becomes a problem, however, when we fail to manage it well, especially the stress that results from problems, frustrations, overwork and worry.

When we don't handle stress well, the body's defences break down and we become susceptible to illness and disease. It's been estimated that over seventy-five percent of all illness is stress-related.Reflexology reduces stress by generating deep, tranquil relaxation. Many clients routinely fall asleep during reflexology sessions and testify on waking that the thirty or forty minutes of sleep were more beneficial and restorative than a full night of restless sleep.

Every part of the body is operated by messages carried back and forth along neural pathways.Stimulation of sensory nerve endings sends information to the spinal cord and brain. The brain and spinal cord send instructions to the organs and muscles. The neural pathways are both living tissueand electrical channels, and can be impinged upon or polluted by many factors. When neural pathways are impaired, nerve function is impeded, messages are delivered slowly and unreliably, or not at all, and body processes operate at less than optimum levels. The Reflexologist stimulates more than 7,000 nerves when touching the feet, and encourages the opening and clearing of neural pathways.

HOW DOES REFLEXOLOGY WORK

In short, by applying pressure to small areas in the feet called "reflex points". Many of my clients and students ask me how does applying pressure to sensitive reflex areas in the feet relieve pain or stimulate an organ. Well, to start with, these reflex areas are only the size of pinheads, so the accuracy of the therapist in detecting these areas and working on them is of paramount importance.No gadgets or "aids" are necessary. In fact, I agree totally with my teacher Ann Gillanders in Great Britain, in saying that we feel that one of the greatest "sins" one can commit is to use probes or electrical stimulating devices as an alternative to using your hands. Hands are ideal for healing, but in order to become a proficient therapist you need to have a genuine compassion for those who suffer, backed by a good basic knowledge of the working of the human body, and the acceptance that you cannot become a reflexologist overnight!. It would also help to understand that it takes time to get results from treatment sessions, just as it took some time to become ill. All too frequently therapists talk to me about clients that expect an instant miracle on their first appointment!.

It is generally considered that Reflexology has the ability to flush out the tissues and improve the circulation, rendering the joints more flexible, stimulating the nervous system and returning the body back to balance.

Dr Fitzgerald also found that if pressure was applied upon the fingers, it could create a local anaesthetic effect from the hand, right up the arm and into the face, ears and nose. He applied the pressure by using special bands of elastic on the middle section of each finger, or small clamps which he placed upon the tips. By this method of anaesthesia he was able to carry out a few minor surgical operations. This finding has similarities to the operations that have been undertaken in recent years,where the only means of anaesthesia used was acupuncture needles which, when placed in the correct position, created a local anaesthetic effect to the organ or area being operated on.

Nature intended that healing should be simple, unfortunately, through the ages man has tried to change this, possibly in ignorance or through a selfish desire for power over others. Most Holistic Natural therapies that have survived to this present time, have grown and are still around becausethey work, if they didn't, then why have they stood the test of time ? Nature has provided a thorough stock of naturally growing remedies to assist. These were provided to help man find some relief from his health problems. But it would seem that we are bent on destroying these self-same remedies including herbs, roots and shrubs. We are also polluting our air and water, so it is not too surprising to realize that our health as a Nation is going to get worse.

When we lump these destructive elements together with a topping of high powered living, which involves tension, worry, frustration and the fight to possess more and more material goods, it is difficult to imagine how mankind will survive at all.

What I feel is missing in the conventional approach to health today is "touch". Most problems treated by doctors are solved with bottles of pills, and I believe I may be right in saying that it is on all too infrequent occasions that doctors examine patients and achieve little if any contact at all. The treatment of disease can be very mechanical; look at the arsenal of mechanical medical equipment at their disposal; doesn't it sometimes take on the appearance of a medieval torture chamber? Even simple devices can look terrifying, like, monitoring machines, X-ray, radiotherapy and chemotherapy, and so on, all of which must create some fear in the patient, not to mention a sometimes cold and clinical approach to suffering.

Because disease is an integral part of the human condition, there is no possible way we can totally eliminate it from our lives. Humans evolve through periods of both health and sickness, and we learn from both. We see sickness as bad and we attack it by means of powerful and often harmful drugs. Any hint of discomfort calls for an immediate visit to the doctor for a prescription. Most often doctors and drugs only serve to make illness less painful. The body sometimes has its own way of coping with these physical imbalances, and drugs often prolong or interfere with the body's healing process. Modern medicine is sometimes preoccupied with getting rid of or masking symptoms. Holistic therapy, on the other hand, can often work quite well with conventional medicine by exploring the cause that the overworked Doctors just don't seem to be able to find the time to do.

This holistic health philosophy considers the body as a dynamic energy system which, like nature, isin a constant state of change. Human beings are more than just their bodies. Each individual is a complex balance of mental, physical and spiritual aspects that are integrated into, and affected directly by, the environment and social problems. The cause of illness is sometimes far more deeply rooted than the symptoms indicate.

Methods
- British School of Reflexology Method
- Reflexology Association of Canada Method
- International School of Reflexology Method
- The Ingham method
- The Colin Paddon Technique

The different methods have been taught to the author and having learned and practised all these modalities I have developed the "Colin Paddon technique", I say this with my tongue-in-cheek almost as a joke. But having said that, I am also serious, because amalgamating the best of each technique and also practising this technique and fine tuning it for many years, has led me to the final technique and homunculus theory of foot reflex points.

The Three Golden Rules To Reflexology
These are very simple rules to follow:

     1. It must do good.
     2. It must feel good.
     3. It must look good.

For obvious reasons "it must do good" is the first rule, if your going to do a treatment you want it tobe productive and beneficial to the client. It doesn't matter how many qualifications you have if its not working. "It must feel good" is the second rule because many people have the mind set that "there's no gain without pain", well, this kind of thinking in reflexology will lose you clients. There is a fine line between "its uncomfortable", and "ouch! that hurts". Working within the boundaries of the pain threshold is the objective. It should be slightly uncomfortable without hurting if its going to do any good. The last aspect of "it must look good" is the results of professionalism, you need to look like you know what your doing, the placement of the hands is important because if the hand positioning looks comfortable and tidy as well as looking relaxed then the client will be more inclined to relax too.

Relaxation Methods

APPLICATION OF CATERPILLAR TECHNIQUE

Caterpillar technique is accomplished by using the outer edge of the thumb. To find this spot, place your hand on the table, palm downwards, you will notice that the edge of the tip of the thumb touches the surface. This is the part of the thumb that you will use to work with on the foot. Caterpillar technique consists of bending the thumb at the first joint so that the thumb takes very small steps along the foot, maintaining equal pressure on the foot at all times. Apply leverage with the other four fingers behind the foot and let the thumb walk along as if pushing down imaginary pins into the skin.

FOOT RELAXATION TECHNIQUES

1. **Diaphragm relaxation**

   With your thumb pressed firmly on the diaphragm line, work medial tolateral and then lateral to medial. Pull the toes and the top of the feet onto the thumb, do not push the thumb into the diaphragm line.

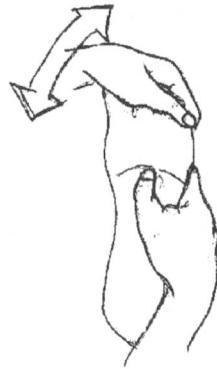

2. **Metatarsal spreading**

   Make a fist with your lateral hand and place this against the ball of the sole of the foot.

   Place the other hand firmly on the dorsal aspect with the thumb covering the toes on the underside. First push with the fist and then pull with the other hand. Alternate this movement to achieve relaxation, first by pushing or spreading the metatarsals and then by closing the other hand slightly and squeezing the foot as you pull back towards yourself.

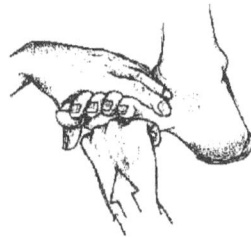

3. **Cushioning**

   With the palm of both hands sandwiching the metatarsals, begin with a slow cycling movement of the hand, whilst gently pushing or cushioning the hands together with the feet between them.

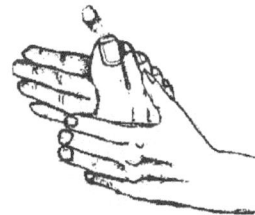

Foot relaxation techniques continued...

4. Ankle freeing

Position your hands, palms over the ankle bones, gently with wrist motion only cause the foot to rock from side to side.

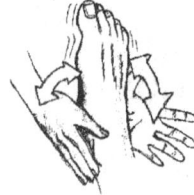

5. Side to side

Place your thumbs on the sole of the foot and your fingers draped over the dorsal aspect of the foot. First push with one hand and pull with the other, then repeat with the other hand.

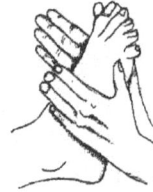

CLIENT CARE

Your client should be seated comfortably supported, preferably seated semi-reclined. Being fully supported is important, if your client wants to relax but has to support their own head then they willbe at a disadvantage and not be able to relax fully. The more they can relax the more effective the treatment will be.

Systematic Treatment Procedure

REFLEXOLOGY TREATMENT ORDER OF WORK

1. Five relaxation techniques:
   a. Diaphragm relaxation
   b. Metatarsal stretching
   c. Cushioning
   d. Ankle freeing
   e. Side to side

2. Sinus area (up)

3. Chronic neck (down)

4. Eyes & ears (rotate)

5. Lung (up)

6. Shoulder (up)

7. Abdominal area (diagonal)

8. Bladder and Kidney (up)

9. Pelvic area (sideways)

10. Spine (up)

11. Hip and Knee (5th met pyramid)

12. Chest and Ribs (reinforced finger)

13. Vas deferens / Fallopian tubes (ankle, both sides two fingers)

14. Prostate / Uterus - Testis / Ovary (both sides)

15. Sciatic area (both sides)

16. Lymph drainage (up the leg lightly)

17. Relaxation techniques

18. Solar plexus with breathing (in-push, out-pull)

ORDER OF WORK

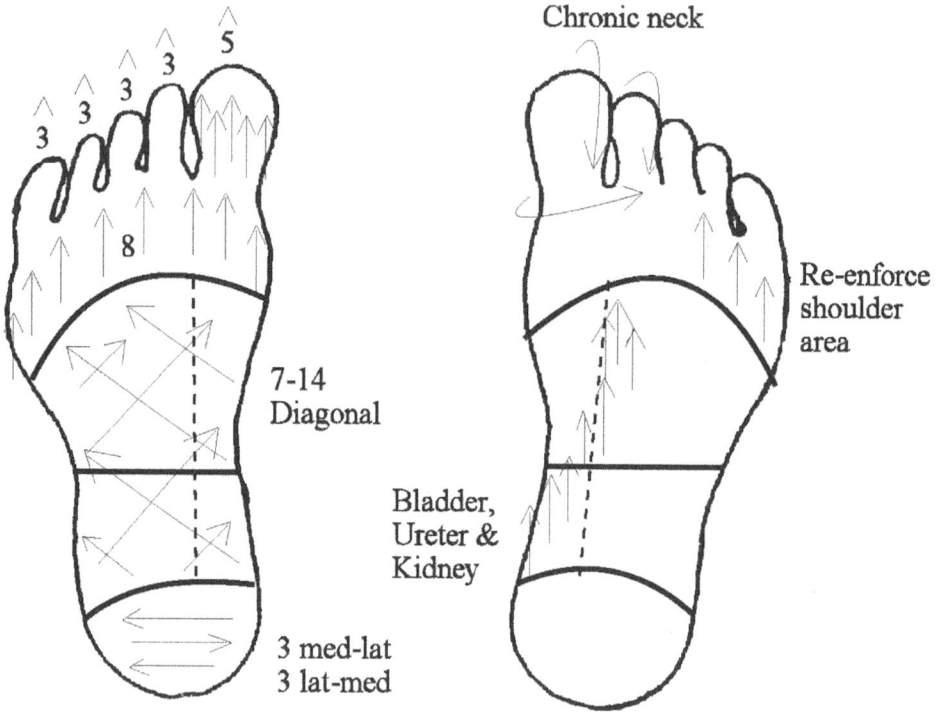

7-14
Diagonal

3 med-lat
3 lat-med

Chronic neck

Re-enforce
shoulder
area

Bladder,
Ureter &
Kidney

REFLEXOLOGY CHART
Reflex Areas

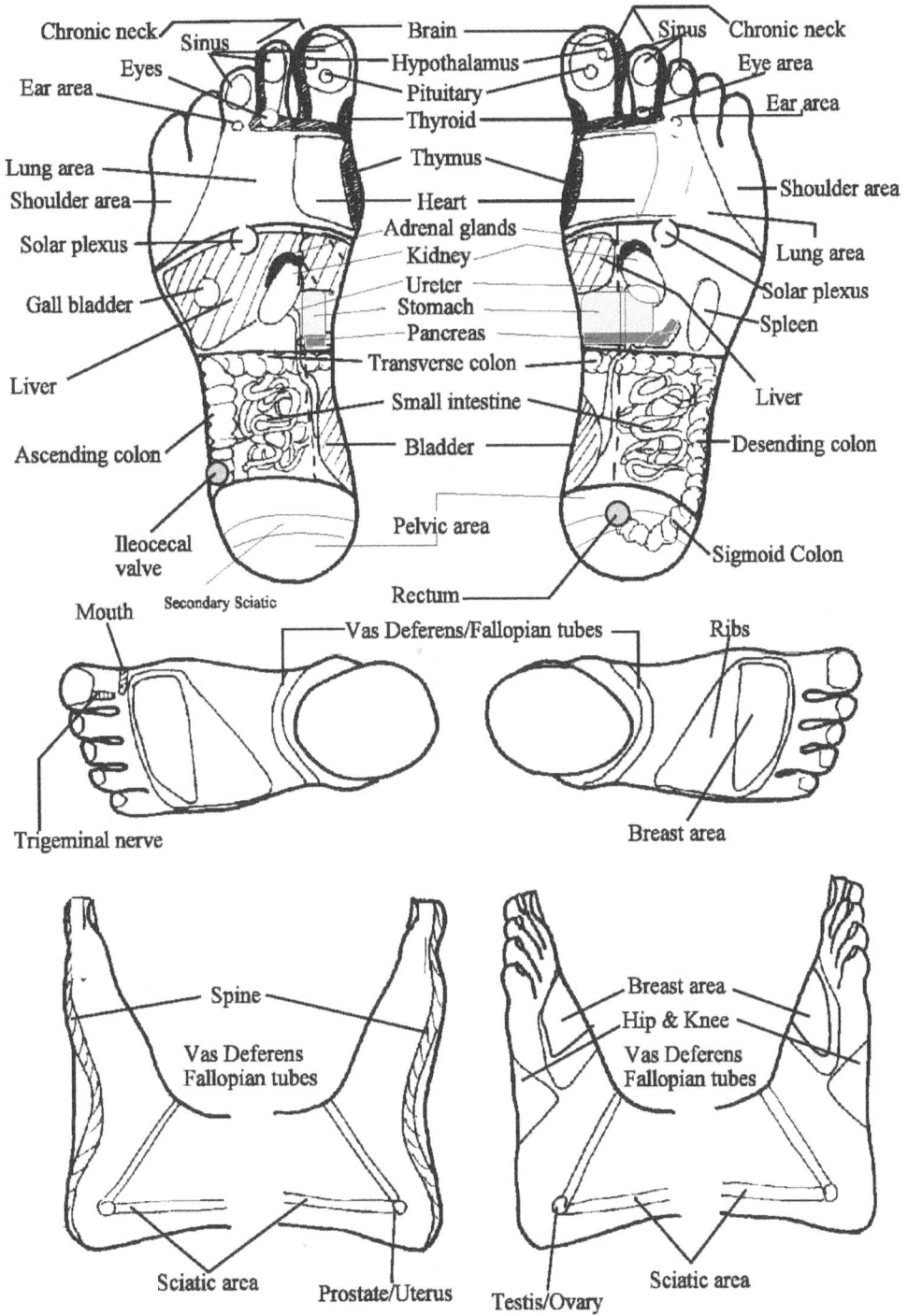

Chronic neck — Sinus — Brain — Sinus — Chronic neck

Eyes — Hypothalamus — Eye area

Ear area — Pituitary — Ear area

Thyroid

Thymus

Lung area — Heart — Shoulder area

Shoulder area — Adrenal glands

Solar plexus — Kidney — Lung area

Ureter — Solar plexus

Gall bladder — Stomach — Spleen

Pancreas

Transverse colon

Liver — Small intestine — Liver

Ascending colon — Bladder — Desending colon

Ileocecal valve — Pelvic area — Sigmoid Colon

Secondary Sciatic — Rectum

Mouth — Vas Deferens/Fallopian tubes — Ribs

Trigeminal nerve — Breast area

Spine — Breast area

Hip & Knee

Vas Deferens Fallopian tubes — Vas Deferens Fallopian tubes

Sciatic area — Prostate/Uterus — Testis/Ovary — Sciatic area

71

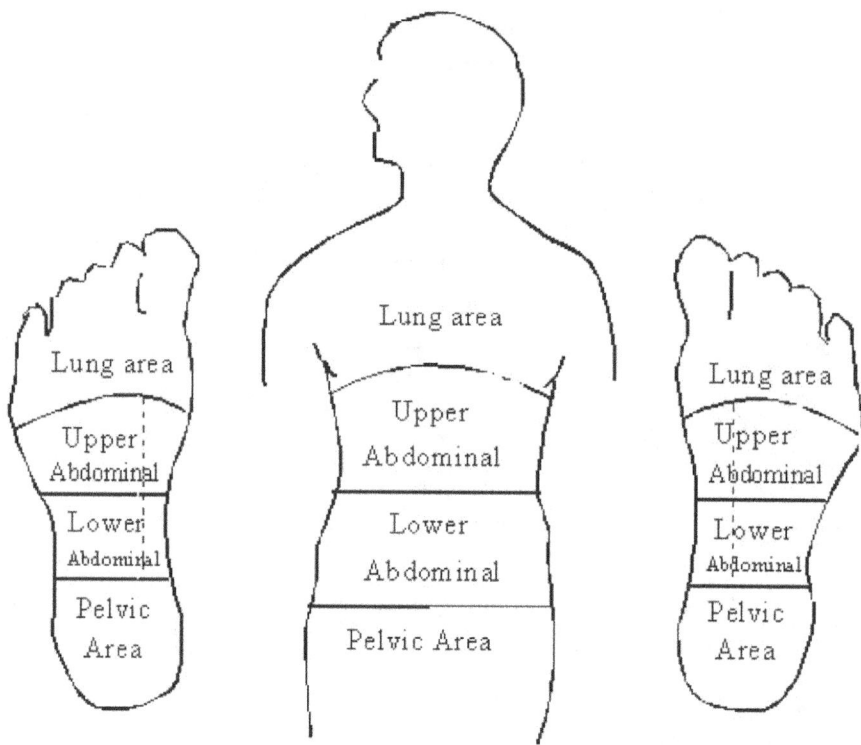

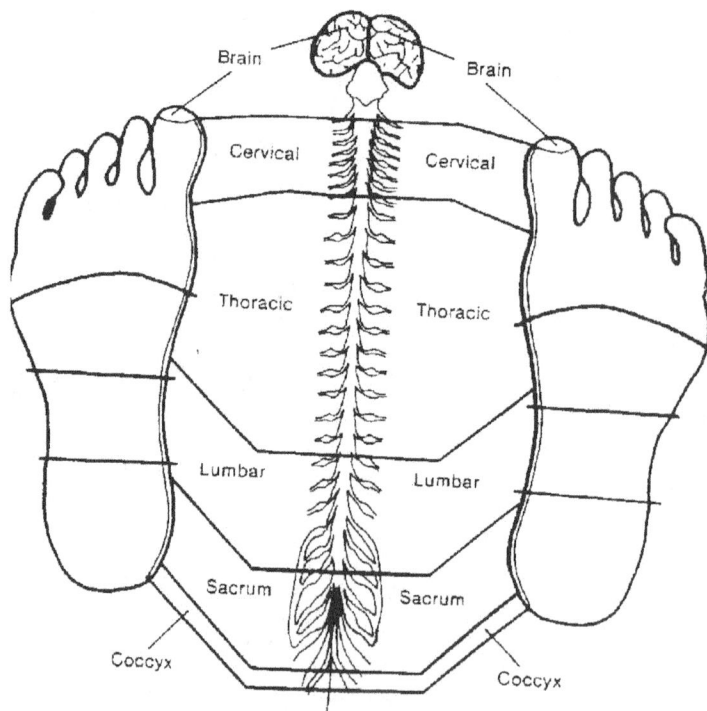

PRACTICE CHART

please feel free to photocopy this chart and practice labelling the reflex areas yourself

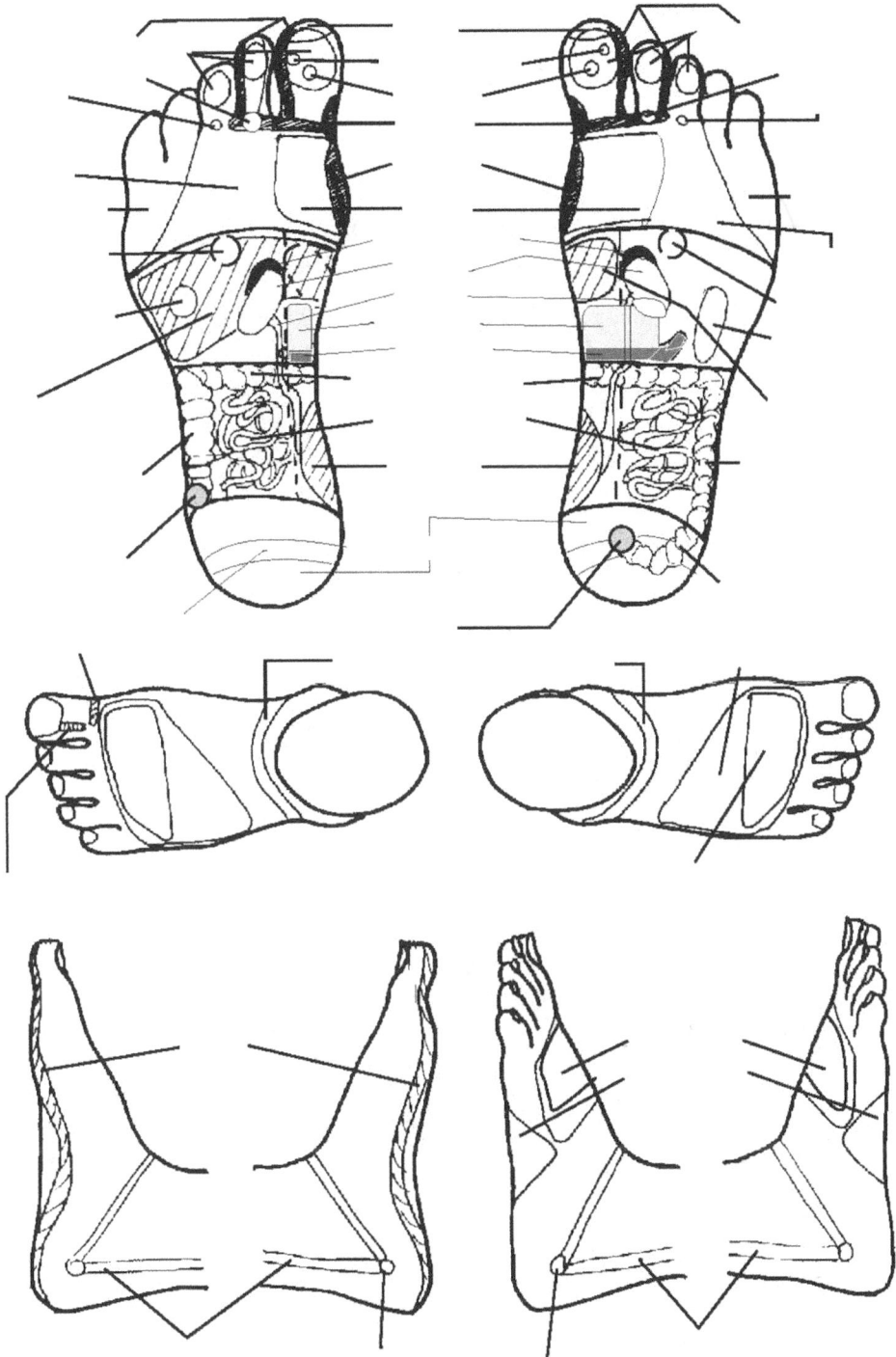

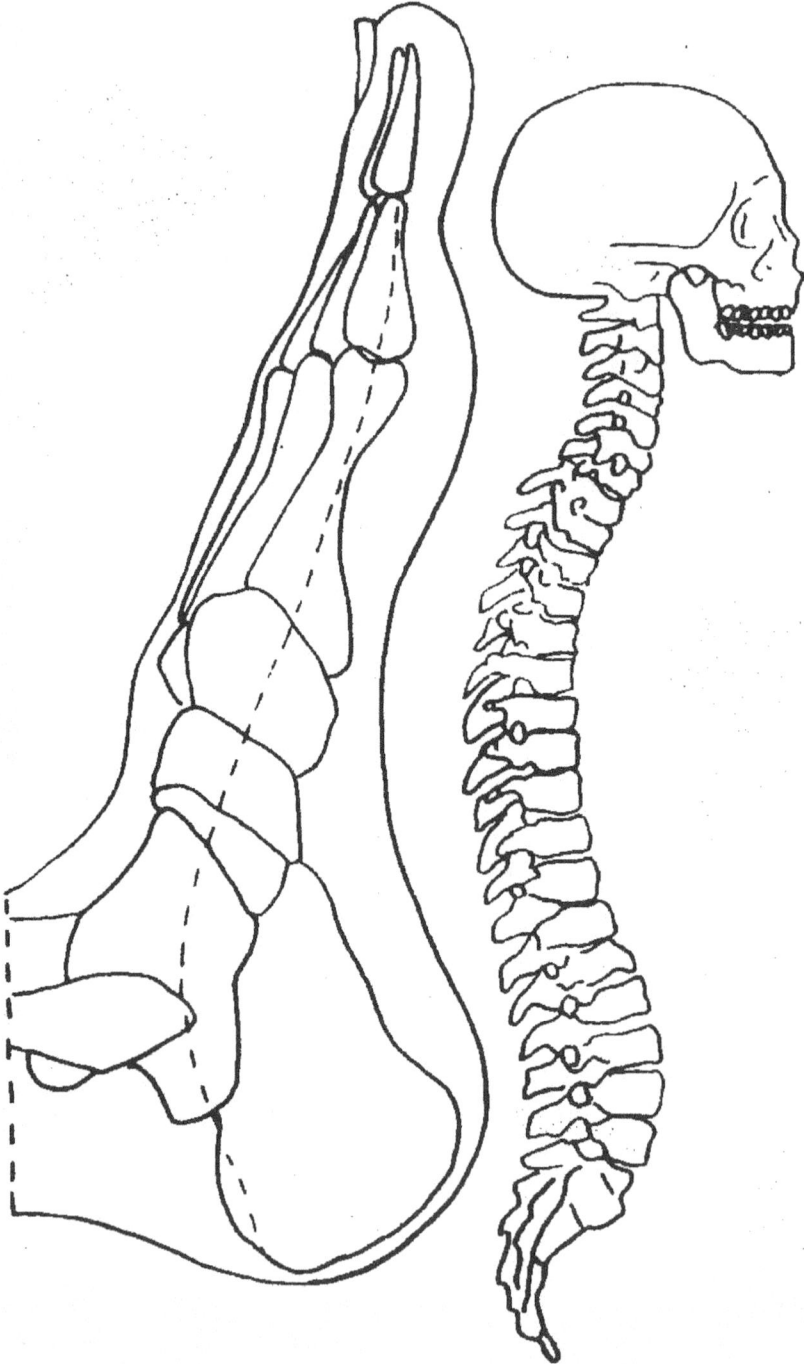

GENITO-URINARY SYSTEM

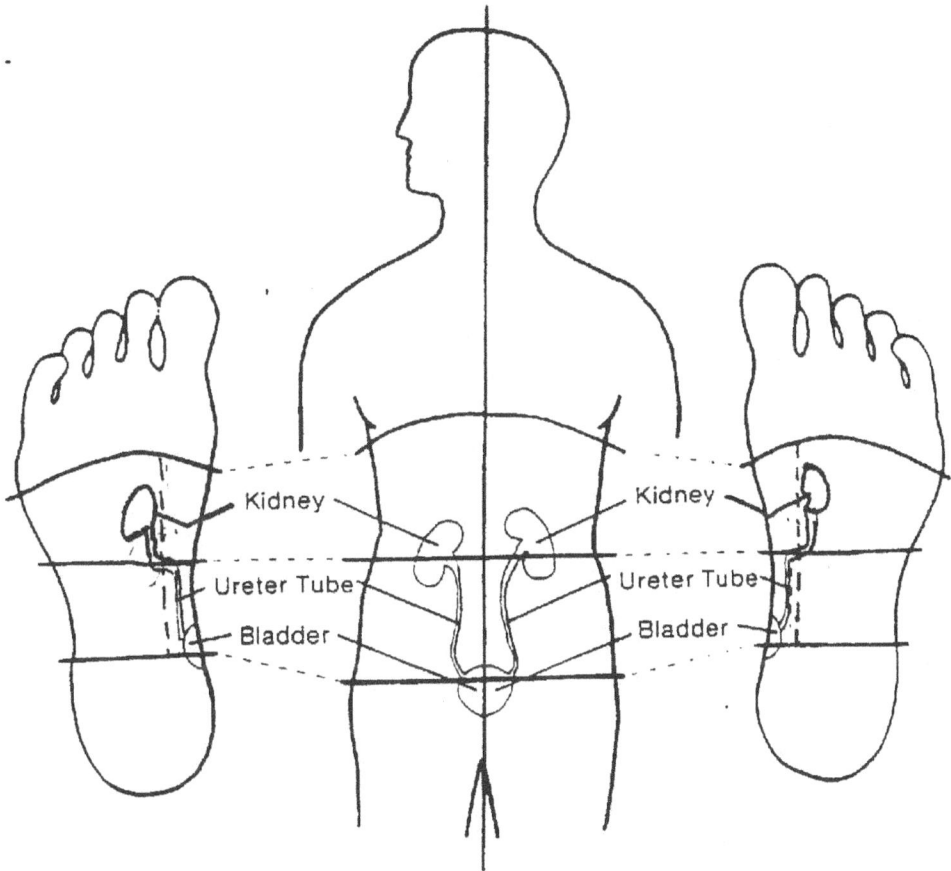

Kidney

Kidney

Ureter Tube

Ureter Tube

Bladder

Bladder

CARDIO-VASCULAR SYSTEM

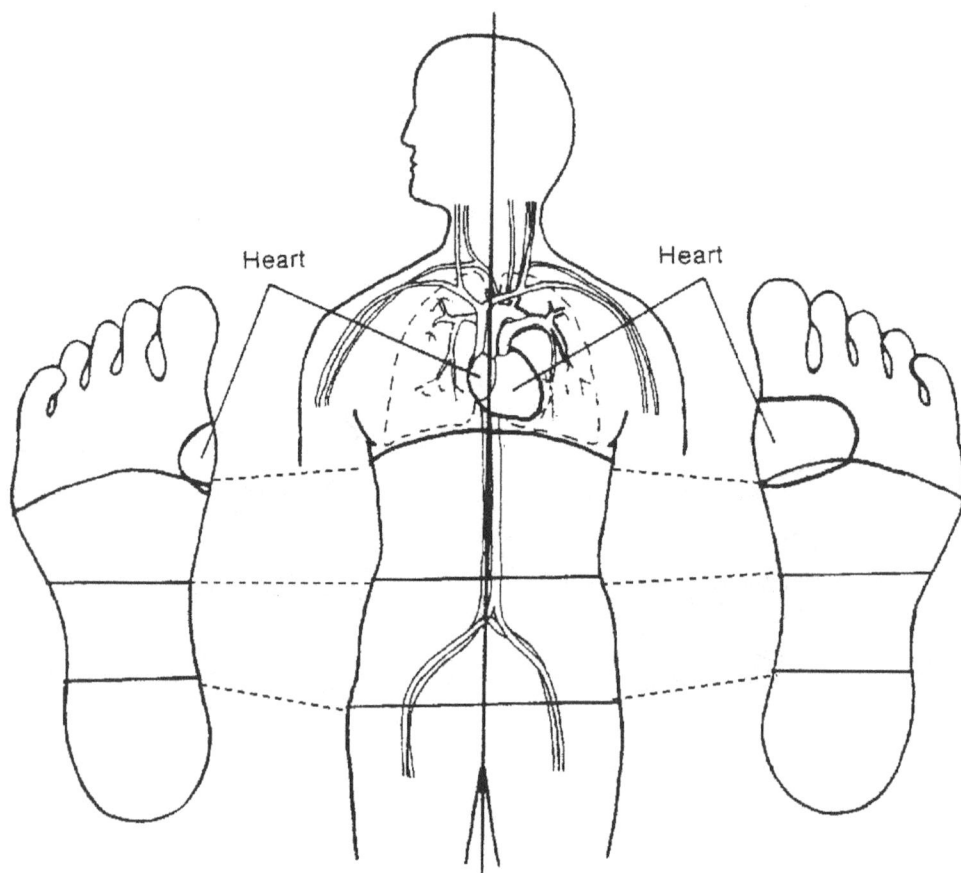

Heart

Heart

MALE or FEMALE REPRODUCTIVE SYSTEM

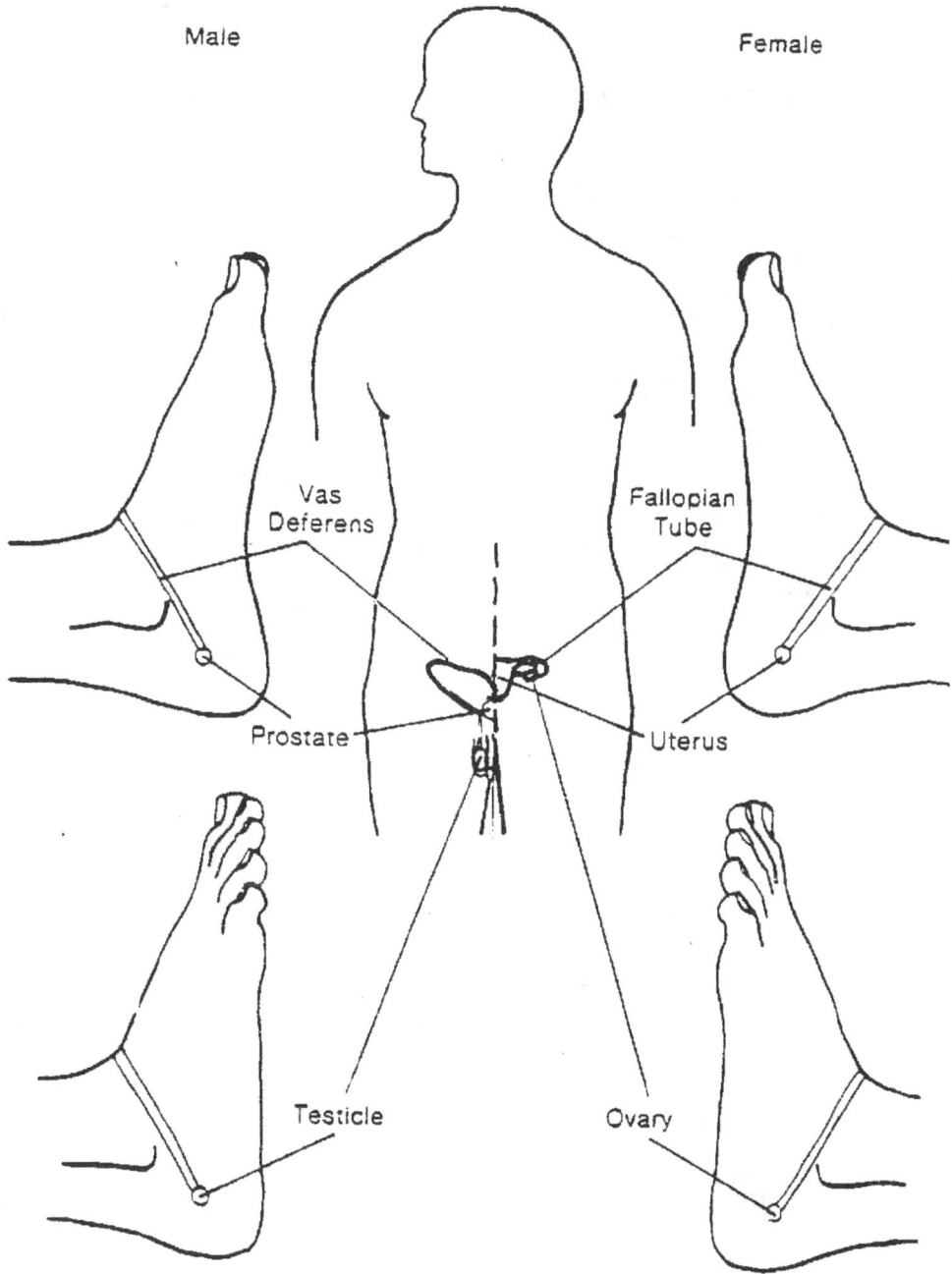

Male

Female

Vas
Deferens

Fallopian
Tube

Prostate

Uterus

Testicle

Ovary

Case-studies and Record-keeping

The following pages contain all the requirements for completing a case-study. These requirements will also help you to assess the problems with your client and to successfully keep records that willhelp you in your practice.

REFLEXOLOGY STUDENT CLIENT RECORD SHEET FOR CASE STUDIES

Therapist	Date	Case Number
Your name goes in here	*First visit with month as 3 letters*	*Numerically expressed*

Client's Name

The client's full name is entered here

Client's Address

The client's full postal address is entered here

D.O.B. clients date of birth / month in 3 letters	*Tel: telephone number here, inc. area code*

All month dates should be entered as a three letter word, ie. Jan, Feb, Mar, etc.

Occupation Job title *State if their job causes them to be active (mobile) or inactive*

Medical History	Medication
Enter all medical information here, regarding hospitalization and ask if they have consulted a doctor about their problem.	*Enter all medication taken here. Enter all vitamins or diet supplements taken as well as allergies etc.*

Medical History: Enter here all relevant information regarding the medical history that the clientwishes to share with you. This information will also help you to build up the overall picture of the clients health problems. Ask questions eg: When was the last time you were in hospital? What was it for? What was the result? And does it effect you now? Repeat these questions again until you have exhausted the hospital history. Also ask, when was the last time you visited your doctor? What was it for? What was the result? And does it effect you now? Repeat these questions again until you have exhausted the visits that are relevant to their personal medical history with their doctor.

Exam p le :	**Medical History:** Hyst 69 GB 73 Thyroidectomy 98	**Medication:** Tylenol 3, Valium Prozac, estrogen RT

Hysterectomy performed in 1969, Gall Bladder removed in 1973, and etc.Use short form that is consistent throughout all the case studies.

Medication:
List all medication and at some later time refer to your books on prescribed drugs to learn about the side effects if any. All too often people come complaining about a health problem and the source could be the side effects experienced with new drugs. Also the information on the drugs as described will also give you a clearer picture into the health problems experienced by the client.

Ask the following questions:

Headaches	sev x 3 pm	Stress level	High Medium Low
Sleep	int x 2	Reproductive	Pregnant Y or No
Bowel	2 pd	Digestive	4 main food groups Yes or No

Headaches: Do you suffer from headaches?
If yes, how often, how severe? What makes them come and what makes them go? Would you consider them mild, moderate or severe?
Sev = severe, Mig = migrain, Mld = mild, X = number of times experienced. Int = interrupted, pd = per day, pw = per week, pm = per month, pa = per annum.

Sleep: How do you sleep? Do you have interrupted sleep? What causes the interruption? Do you wake up tired? Do you have trouble getting off to sleep?
Int x 2 = two interruptions during the night for what ever reason.

Bowel: Are you regular? Are you more prone to going too often or not enough?
pd = per day, pw = per week

Digestive: Are you eating the four main food groups? Are you drinking enough water? Do you have problems digesting fats? Do you have any food allergies? Do you suffer from any gas, bloating or stomach pain?

Reproductive: Are you pregnant? Is there any possibility that you might be pregnant? Are there any problems with your reproductive system that you know of?

General Health: How would you describe your general health today? Do you feel that your energy level is high or low?

Contra-indications: Have you suffered or do you suffer from any of the following; TB, HIV, epilepsy, hepatitis, dermatitis, high or low blood pressure, or any thing else that you would like to tell me? If they answer "Yes" ask them if they would like to disclose any information?

The remainder of the chart is completed by observation and body analysis, during the practical examination and assessment of the client.

Do not leave any blank or unanswered questions/boxes.
Do not check ✓ or similar representation, it does not offer information.
Write N/A = not applicable where needed, do not cross out options.

REFLEXOLOGY STUDENT
CLIENT RECORD SHEET FOR CASE STUDIES

Reason for clients visit/what are you treating/Desired effect

Therapist _____ Date _____

Case Number _____

Client's Name in full _____

Client's Address _____

D.O.B. _____ Tel: _____

Occupation: _____

Medical History

Medication

Vitamins

Headaches	Spleen
Sleep	Stomach
Bowel	Kidneys
Eating habits	Bladder
Reproductive	Colon
Stress	Ileocecal
Sinus	Sigmoid
Shoulders	Sciatic
Eyes	Prostate/Testis
Ears	Uterus/Ovary
Chronic neck	Pelvis
Lungs	Vas deferens/fallopian
Heart	knee/hip
Liver	Chest
Gall bladder	Face

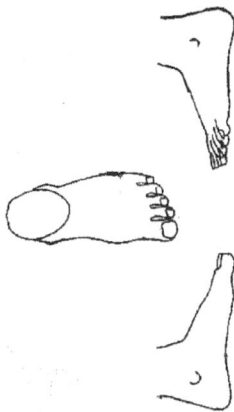

1. This is to acknowledge that I have been informed about the Reflexology treatment being offered and I fully understand and accept that this treatment is being performed by a student Reflexologist.

2. I also agree to this information being stored and used as part of the mandatory case studies required by the above student.

3. I do not wish to have this personal information given to any other person or business and I understand that I may be contacted at some time from the school to verify that I did in fact receive a treatment from the above named student.

4. I also understand that the Reflexologist performing this treatment is not a medical doctor, nor is he/she diagnosing, prescribing or replacing my family doctor.

signed:_____ date:_____

Reflexology for Holistic Therapists

Essential Oils and Creams

TI-TREE (TEA TREE)
Latin name: *melaleuca alternifolia*   **Botanical family**: *Myrtaceae*

The three main areas where this oil can help are:
1. Auto-immune system stimulant
2. Colds, influenza, viral infections
3. Strong anti-septic/anti-fungal for nails and skin care

PROPERTIES	USES
Antiviral	Influenza, warts, herpes, cold sores
Antifungal	Candida, athlete's foot, thrush, yeast infections, fungal infections,genital warts
Antiseptic	Cystitis, urinary tract infections, skin care, boils, acne, mouthulcers, gum infections
Immunostimulant	Infections, debility, infectious diseases

Place of Origin
This tree is primarily a native of Australia. It is a member of the Myrtacaceae family as eucalyptus and clove. It is a relative new comer to the Aromatherapy field, yet highly regarded for its diversified uses.

Method of Extraction
The essential oil of ti-tree is distilled from the leaves of the plant. The main chemical constituents include: terpineol with various alcohols and monoterpenes. The oil may be colourless to a pale yellow hue with a distinctive medicinal odor.

Traditional Uses
The Aborigines in Australia have used the plant to help heal wounds. It was introduced to the European countries in the late 1920's and was used in first aid kits by the military in World War 2. Today, many products are using ti-tree in deodorants, toothpastes, skin care produces and more for its versatile nature.

Herbal Medicine
Tea tree has been used in dermatological conditions such as acne vulgaris

Reflexology

Tea tree has a wide range of uses in the reflexology field. This is due to the fact that it is antiviral, antifungal and antibacterial in nature.

It has been proven to be a very powerful immune system stimulant. It does this by activating the white blood cells to fight off any intruders (virus, bacteria and fungi). Glandular fevers, debility and other debilitating illnesses are indications for treatment with ti-tree. It may possibly be effective for AIDS.

Viral infections from influenza to warts and herpes (both oral and genital) respond to this essential oil. Sprays can be made up to use in infected rooms. The spray is also safe to use in the case of herpes, oryou may wish to apply a drop directly onto the affected area. Warts need an application a minimum of one per day. It may take a few weeks to see results, but it is an effective means of treatment.

Many people today suffer from candida and other yeast infections as well as fungal infections like athletes foot and thrush. Use ti-tree for these problems, but it is important to continue the use of this essence for 1-2 months after the symptoms disappear. Sprays or douches are effective means for treating vaginal yeast infections.

Tea tree may induce perspiration when used to alleviate colds and flu. This is a good sign as it increases the immune response. Most naturopaths believe in allowing a fever to run its course without medication as long as it stays below 104 degrees F. This does not hold true in infants, young children, geriatrics and the chronically ill. It is important to seek the appropriate medical attention in these cases in order to maintain safety.

Essential oil of ti-tree may be used as a gargle for the treatment of gum diseases. Bad breath or mouth ulcers. Do not swallow.

MYRRH

The three main areas where this oil can help are:
1. Cuts and wounds.
2. Eczema type skin disorders.
3. Mouth infections.

PROPERTIES	USES
Antiseptic	Amenorrhoea Pyorrhoea
Antiphlogistic	Aphthae Stomatitis
Astringent	Catarrh Tuberculosis
Carminative	Chlorosis Ulcers-skin & mouth
Emmenagogue	Cough Wounds
Expectorant	Diarrhoea
Sedative	Dyspepsia
Stimulant (especially ulmonary)	Flatulence
Stomachic	Gingivitis
Tonic	Haemorrhoids
Uterine	Leucorrhoea
Vulnerary	Loss of appetite

Place of Origin
Myrrh is a resin produced by a small tough spiny tree which grows in semi-arid regions of Libya, Iran, along the Red Sea, and various Places in North East Africa. it is also found in The "Garden of Eden" which was part of Babylonia in the time of Moses. The tree or shrub, grows only to a height of nine feet, with small white flowers and trifoliate leaves which are also aromatic.

Method of Extraction
The liquid resin is exuded from natural cracks or cuts in the trunk of the tree, and sets into irregularly shaped brownish-red lumps. As with Frankincense, modern harvesting consists of making systematic cuts in wild trees, and to an extent, cultivated trees.

The essential oil is extracted from the resin by steam distillation, and is a deep reddish-brown and may need warming before it is possible to pour it from the bottle. It has a smoky aromatic smell.

The active principles include: pinene, dipentene, limonene, cadinene, formic acid, acetic acid, myrrholic acid, eugenol, several aldehydes and alcohols, and a number of resins.

In common with Frankincense, Myrrh was used in all the ancient civilisations as a perfume, incense and in medicine. It was highly valued as a healing ointment for wounds and it is said that no soldier ofAncient Greece went into battle without a paste of Myrrh in his pouch. This use is well justified by what we know of Myrrh's antiseptic, healing and anti-inflammatory properties. Myrrh is especially valuable for wounds that are slow to heal or for weepy skin conditions.

Eczema and athlete's foot respond to Myrrh, the fungicidal constituent sees to that. It will also heal cracked and chapped skin.

Myrrh is very good for gums, and quickly heals mouth ulcers and most gum disorders. The most convenient method is to use myrrh in the mouth as a tincture. It will sting and taste bitter (awful), but the healing effects are well worth the initial discomfort or inconvenience. It is used in many brands of tooth paste with essential oil of peppermint to mask its bitterness and to make it palatable.

Chest infections like, catarrh, chronic bronchitis, colds and sore throats, respond well to inhalations of myrrh. It is a good pulmonary antiseptic, expectorant and astringent. Best used in a massage oil or inhalations as it is very difficult to dissolve, even in alcohol.

Some care should be considered when using myrrh, as it is emmenagogic and should not be used during pregnancy.

Myrrh has a tonic and stimulating action on the stomach and in fact the whole digestive tract, and is a remedy for diarrhoea.

Because of the antifungal action of myrrh, it can be used in a vaginal douche against thrush. It will eliminate the itch and discharge effectively, but thought should also be given to the underlying candida infection which leads to these symptoms, and ti-tree oil, with perhaps a special diet used.

LEMON

Latin Name: *citrus Limonium*   **Botanical name**: *Rutaceae*

The three main areas where this oil can help are:

1. Circulatory problems
2. Immune stimulant
3. Wounds and cuts

PROPERTIES	USES
Tonic	Circulatory system, varicose veins, chilblains, broken capillaries, arteriosclerosis, digestive system
Anti-viral/Immunostimulant	Influenza, respiratory infection, colds, catarrh, warts
Haemostatic	Cuts, nosebleeds, bleeding gums
Antiseptic	Infections, bronchitis, asthma, oily skin, pimples, acne

Place of Origin
The lemon tree is thought to have originated in India, and to have been introduced into Italy towards the end of the 5th Century. From Italy, cultivation spread throughout the Mediterranean basin to Spain and Portugal. California now rivals the traditional growing area in commercial terms.

Method of Extraction
The essential oil of lemon is pressed from the outer rind of the lemons. It takes as many as 3,000 of them to produce a kilo of essential oil. The oil is a pale yellow colour with a hint of green and obviously smells like the fresh clean scent of lemon. Its active constituents include pinene, limonene, phellandrene, camphene, linalol, acetates of linalol and geranyl, citral and citrinellal.

Traditional Uses
A plant dating back in history, it arrived in Europe during the Crusades. Long used for its antiseptic abilities, it has been used during infectious epidemics. The peel has known to be used to scent clothing as well as utilized as an insect repellant.
It was in the 17th Century that it was discovered to be valuable for its "medicinal" use (due to the high Vitamin C content) for infection and toxicity.

Herbal Uses

Lemon juice, especially first thing in the morning is an excellent digestive aid that will increase thedigestive juices while cleansing and decongesting the liver. Also known for its cleansing abilities on the blood, it has been used as a styptic to help stop blood flow.

Reflexology

Similar to the herbal uses, lemon has a tonifying and stimulating action on many systems. Through the use of this essential oil, the digestive system will find a reduction in gastric acidity. It can be used in cases of debility and loss of appetite, but its main use in Reflexology is to apply Essential Lemon oil directly onto a wart, this will diminish the wart in size until it disappears altogether.

Lemon will stimulate both gastric and pancreatic secretions. (It has been used in the treatment of diabetes). The liver and kidneys will also benefit from the detoxifying and cleansing action of this essential oil.

Lemon possesses a unique ability to counteract acidity in the body even though the nature of lemon is acidic. However, the citric acid is neutralised during the digestion process. It will increase the carbonates and bi-carbonates of potassium and calcium and these in turn will help maintain the alkalinityof the system. Ulcers or cases where there is an imbalance in the acid/alkaline balance will find improvement. These disorders include problems where there is an excess of uric acid in the system such as gout, rheumatism, arthritis, etc. To further assist the elimination of internal uric acid, it would be wise to bath in 1 cup of dead sea salts, or epsom salts three times per week. The alkaline nature of these salts help disperse the acid build up found in the joints.

A powerful antiseptic, essential oil of lemon can be used for the treatment of colds, bronchitis, catarrh and in the prevention of infectious diseases. Lemon is a powerful bactericide which is another excellent reason to use it in the treatment of cuts. Dr. Jean Valnet cites research which has shown that essential oil will kill diphtheria bacilli in 20 minutes and even in a low dilution (0.2%). It will render the tuberculosis bacilli completely inactive.

Furthermore it is an immunostimulant that increases the action of the white blood cells boosting the body's immune response to viruses and other immune disorders.

Haemostatic in nature, nosebleeds, minor cuts and wounds, and bleeding gums will benefit from its styptic properties. Bleeding gums, gingivitis or mouth ulcers will improve with the utilization of a mouthwash. For nosebleeds, soak a small piece of cotton into some lemon juice and insert it into the nostril.

Lemon has a tonic effect on the circulatory system and finds a use for varicose veins, arteriosclerosis,broken capillaries, high blood pressure and chilblains. Regular use improves sluggish circulation, byreducing blood viscosity and helps break down any hardened deposits.

Warning: Possible skin irritant. As with most citrus oils, lemon is photo toxic. UV lighting (the sun or sun bed) should be avoided after use of this essence.

RECIPES FOR FOOT CARE

Diffuser blend recipes....

Calming and Uplifting	Antiseptic	To Promote Sleep
2 drops Lavender	1 drop Pine	1 drop Lavender
1 drop Ylang Ylang	2 drops Eucalyptus	1 drop Chamomile
1 drop Rose	1 drop Ti-Tree	1 drop Clary Sage
Allergies/Sinus	**Meditation**	**Stimulating**
Congestion	1 drop Frankincense	2 drops Rosemary
3 drops Eucalyptus	1 drop Clary Sage	1 drop Basil
1 drop Camphor	1 drop Hyssop	1 drop Grapefruit
Asthmatic blend	**Antiseptic blend**	**Morning Wake-Up Call**
2 drops of Eucalyptus	4 drops of Ti-tree	4 drops of Lemon
1 drop of Chamomile	1 drop of Lemon	2 Drops of Rosemary
	Mix into one teaspoon	1 drop of Orange
	of VodkaTop-up with	1 drop of Rose
	125ml Distilled water	

Specific usage...

Cuts	Burns	Fungus on nails
Place 1-2 drops of Myrrh without diluting it or adding anything to it, directly onto the wound. Repeat two to three times a day	Place a few drops of undiluted Lavender directly onto the burn, the pain will subside very soon	Place one drop of Ti-tree directly on the nail and repeat twice a day until it is gone

Bath blend recipes...

Relaxing, Uplifting Bath	Stimulating Morning Bath	Foot Bath for Tired Feet
2 drops Lavender	2 drops Peppermint	1 drop Lavender
2 drops Chamomile	2 drops Rosemary	1 drop Peppermint
1 drop Ylang Ylang	2 drops Juniper	1 drop Lemon
1 drop Patchouli		
Muscular Aches and Pains	**Cellulite Bath**	**Cleansing, Detoxifying Bath**
2 drops Marjoram	2 drops Grapefruit	2 drops Lemon
2 drops Black Pepper	2 drops Juniper	2 drops Juniper
2 drops Lavender	2 drops Cypress	2 drops Geranium

Creams

Hypo-allergenic cream bases derived from natural sources are the best medium to mix essential oils into. Carrier oils are just as effective. These creams or carrier oils can be customized to suit any problem from headaches, sinus infections or problems with skin care, aches and pains etc. These creams can then be applied to the affected area to help alleviate the existing problem.

Recipes...

Headache Cream	Sinus Cream
3 drops Peppermint 3 drops Lavender 30 ml Base Cream	2 drops Eucalyptus 2 drops Camphor 1 drop Peppermint 30 ml Base cream If an infection is present versus just congestion, then 2 drops of ti-treecan be used as well.
Aches and Pains	Skin Care
3 drops Marjoram 2 drops Black Pepper 2 drops Lavender 30 ml Base Cream	3 drops Lavender 3 drops Geranium 3 drops Roman Chamomile (1 drop if using German Chamomile) In 30 ml Base Cream 10 drops oil of Evening Primrose

Poultices and Compresses

Compresses can draw out impurities from the skin, help soothe any irritation, pain and/or infection present. They are an old and very good method of applying oils to a specific area of the body. They can be done either hot or cold. A hot compress should be as hot as possible. These are used to reduce muscular and rheumatic pain, to draw out boils, splinters or infections, to relieve menstrual cramps,toothaches, etc. A cold compress may be used for sprains, swelling, headaches and to reduce fever. If a cold compress is called for, add ice cubes in the water to reduce the temperature further. Compresses can also be used to aid the absorption of essential oil applied with massage to the area of the body requiring treatment. For example, you could apply an expectorant chest rub, then a compress. This will work because the essences are absorbed into the skin even when the temperature of the compress changes.

To make a compress add approximately 4 drops of essential oil to about 1000 ml (1 litre) of water. Saturate the compress by dipping it close to the surface of the water so that much of the floating oil is absorbed into the compress. Squeeze out the excess water. For added effectiveness, an herbal infusion of the same plant can be used instead of water.

Abscesses/Boils	Burns
2 drops Ti-Tree 2 drops Eucalyptus	Apply lavender neat onto the skin. For a analgesic effect, apply a cool compress with: 2 drops Lavender 2 drops Chamomile
Itching and Eczema	**Insect Bites/Poison Ivy**
2 drops Chamomile 1 drop Lavender 1 drop Geranium	2 drops Eucalyptus 1 drop Lavender 1 drop Ti-Tree

Setting Up Your Own Business

The best thing to do would be to work for someone else to get experience in the market and to get yourface known. This is the best way to find out if this kind of life is for you and to get to know all the in-rules in and around your neighbourhood without getting into too much trouble or debt. The secret to success is to never use your own money/savings and to put as much income as you can into your own business, before you pay yourself. If you only want to work certain hours and times, then working for someone else would be the best idea. If you want to work for yourself, be prepared to work long hours with little pay for the long haul and you might succeed.

To work for yourself ask your self what do I have, what do I need and what do I want.

What do I have: List all the things you have now that will help you get into business, this includes money and support as well.

What do I need: List all the things you believe you will need to get into business, but keep it basic. When you have done this, cross off the things you have already and try and put a price to all the things you still need to get.

What do I want: This is the best list of all, because you can let your imagination free to explore the possibilities of how you see yourself as you become more successful.

Draw up a business plan and try to project just how you are going to do this including projections of income and expenditure.

PROFESSIONAL REQUIREMENTS

But lets get back to basics, what do I basically need to get into business for myself?

You will need somewhere to work, like an office or room that you're renting. You will need a reclining chair like a lazy-boy to offer your clients and a small stool to work from. A custom designed aesthetics/beauticians chair would be ideal but they tend to cost in excess of $1000.00 and that might be out of your budget range. Some towels and massage cream with essential oils, and antiseptic soap. You will need a phone and business cards. The best way to get your name out there is not by advertising, but by word of mouth. Start small and get referrals then get your referrals to get more referrals. Place your business card in health food stores and local stores near your practice.

You do not need to charge GST unless you plan on doing excess of $30,000.00 in your first year. Health services are exempt PST. Get a book keeper if you can't do it yourself, and when you are doing better, get an accountant. Start off as a self-employed therapist and if business is good think about incorporating, it will save you a lot of money.

WHAT TO DO NEXT

- Read this book from cover to cover and watch the video many times.
- Practice drawing the reflex points as many times as you need to, until you can do it completely from memory.
- Practice the caterpillar technique until you have perfected it. (Remember, it will hurt/ache until you get it right and build up some muscle).
- Practice on a friend until it begins to feel comfortable and the order of work is coming to you naturally.
- Complete 25 case studies and you will be ready to be assessed.
- When you can draw the foot reflex areas accurately you will be ready to complete the theory exam.

Good luck!

INDEX